BUTEYKO

BREATHING TECHNIQUES

ENCYCLOPEDIA

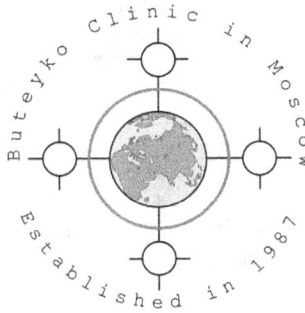

Anna Novozhilova
Claudia Schyia

BUTEYKO

BREATHING TECHNIQUES

ENCYCLOPEDIA

Edited by Dr Andrey E. Novozhilov
Co-author of the Buteyko Method

2025

Published in 2025 by FeedARead.com Publishing

British Library CIP
A CIP catalogue record for this title is available from the British Library.

Disclaimer
This book is presented solely for educational purposes. It is not intended as a substitute for the medical advice of a health professional. The reader should regularly consult a physician in matters relating to his/her health and particularly with respect to any symptoms that may require diagnosis or medical attention. The publisher and authors are not responsible for any specific health needs that may require medical supervision and are not liable for any damages or negative consequences from any treatment, action, application or preparation to any person reading or following the information of this book. Any use of the information in this book is at the reader's discretion. The authors and the publisher specifically disclaim any and all liability arising directly or indirectly from the use or application of any information or instructions contained in this book.

5 PRACTICE classes and theory of
GENUINE Buteyko Breathing Techniques

from
BUTEYKO Clinic in MOSCOW (est. 1987)

Professor Buteyko – New Zealand Conference Dec '00

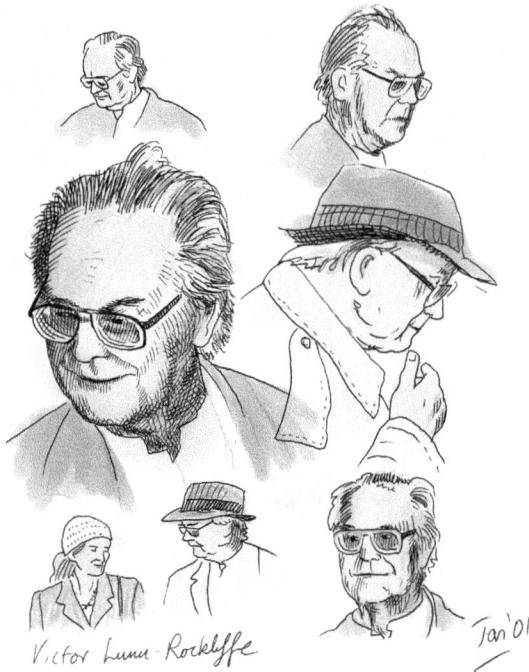

Victor Lunn-Rockliffe

Jan '01

Moscow (Russia) & Cologne (Germany)
2025

In the hope that our joint project will help many people
to return to a healthy life

Authors

Preface

More than half a century has passed since the Russian doctor and scientist Dr Konstantin Pavlovich Buteyko made a fundamental **scientific discovery in medicine** and invented **a drug-free method of treatment**, commonly known as '**the Buteyko Method**'.

In this book, the authors talk about the famous part of the Buteyko Method – about the genuine Buteyko breathing technique, which was invented and applied by the author himself, Dr Buteyko, and which for three generations continues to save the lives of millions of people (without any exaggeration) suffering from bronchial asthma, allergies, high blood pressure and many other diseases.

Leading scientists in various fields of medical science agree that Dr Buteyko **deciphered the secret knowledge of Indian yogis** about **health, Christian ascetics** and the strength of the spirit, and **put this knowledge at the service of us all.**

Nature has given us the ability to control breathing across a wide range, **and Dr Buteyko has taught us how** to measure and normalize breathing in order to maintain and improve health.

This book is primarily a guide for those who have already attended Buteyko courses with a specialist certified by the Buteyko Clinic in Moscow (est. 1987). The reader will find a well-structured handbook which is intended to be helpful for those who are already familiar with the Buteyko breathing technique.

Some repetition of the material in the authors' articles reveals various aspects of Dr Buteyko's difficult and extraordinary scientific discovery and makes the scientific material **simpler and more understandable**.

The practical part of the book is richly illustrated for a better understanding of the material.

At the end of the book there is a **Glossary** with an explanation of technical terms for the Buteyko Method, with explanations by Andrey Novozhilov, MD. For the first time we give a **scientific definition of terms** that are used when describing the Buteyko Method, such as 'Deep breathing', 'The art of ephemeral, imperceptible breathing', or 'The art of reducing the depth of breathing with a light volitional effort', and many others.

Contents

Authors of the articles

Anna Novozhilova, Director of the programme

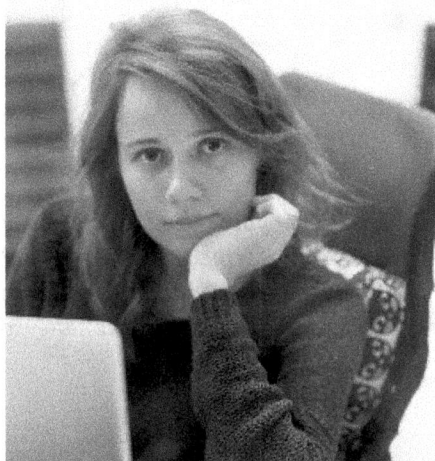

Anna Novozhilova, Director of the programme 'Genuine Buteyko breathing techniques from Primary Sources for Foreigners', Buteyko Clinic in Moscow (est. 1987)

Director of the programme 'Genuine Buteyko breathing techniques from Primary Sources for Foreigners'.

Born in Moscow, she graduated from Moscow State University of International Relations (MGIMO) and then completed a Master's degree at the Universitat Autònoma de Barcelona (UAB).

Since 2015 she is the author, translator and adapter of the original Buteyko programmes in Russian into English and Spanish languages.

She was trained as a Buteyko Method specialist:
- directly by Dr Konstantin P. Buteyko, MD, PhD, author of the Buteyko Method;
- directly by Dr Lyudmila D. Buteyko (Novozhilova), co-author of the Buteyko Method;
- directly by Dr Andrey E. Novozhilov, MD, chief physician of the Buteyko Clinic in Moscow, co-author of the Buteyko Method, copyright holder.

Anna is the goddaughter of Dr Konstantin P. Buteyko.

Claudia Schyia, Certified Specialist

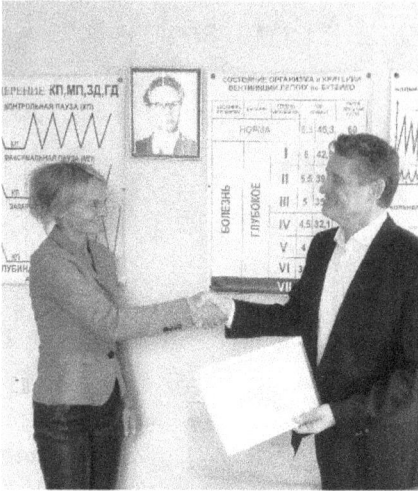

Dr Andrey E. Novozhilov, co-author of the Buteyko Method and copyright holder, presenting *Claudia Schyia* with the Specialist Certificate at the Buteyko Clinic in Moscow

Certified Buteyko Method Specialist, Germany (Cologne)

For 40 years I have been looking for a way to cure bronchial asthma and no longer be dependent on medication. I researched numerous possible treatments, including yoga, proper nutrition, sports, a healthy lifestyle and much more, but asthma did not succumb and did not subside. Medical doctors told me directly and honestly that asthma could not be cured with medication, so this disease was with me for life.

One day I heard about Dr Konstantin P. Buteyko from Russia, who had invented a non-drug way to treat asthma, known as the Buteyko Method. I learned the Buteyko Method and now I've been living for several years without asthma and almost without medication.

Dr Andrey E. Novozhilov, MD, Chief Physician

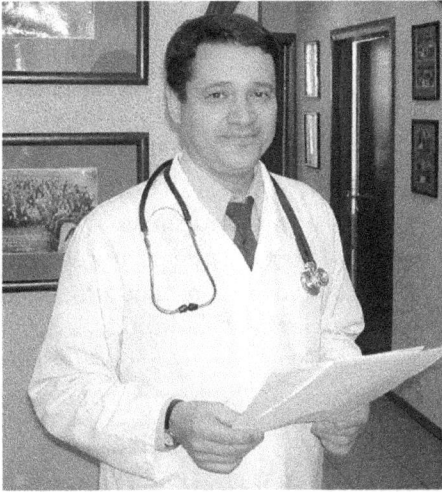

Dr Andrey E. Novozhilov, MD, *chief physician of the Buteyko Clinic in Moscow (est. 1987), in 2005*

Chief physician of the Buteyko Clinic in Moscow, co-author of the Buteyko Method, copyright holder (since 2014).

Born in Moscow and graduate of the Sechenov First Moscow State Medical University with a degree in Medical Science, General Medicine.

Dr Novozhilov became acquainted with the Buteyko Method at the age of 9, when his mother, Lyudmila Buteyko (Novozhilova), twice suffered clinical death as a result of severe asthma suffocation attacks.

Dr Buteyko was invited to treat his mother and assessed her serious condition. He told 9-year-old Andrey how to reduce her breathing in order to cure her bronchial asthma. So the son cured the mother. Two weeks later, the asthma attacks completely stopped.

Since 1989, he has been the chief physician in the Buteyko Clinic. He is the author of a unique programme for the treatment of bronchial asthma which allows former asthmatics to return to active life and cure any form of the disease, regardless of its severity and prescription.

The reference book *Who's Who* includes information about Dr Andrey E. Novozhilov and the medical institution that has been working steadily for more than 20 years.

Dr Lyudmila D. Buteyko (Novozhilova), Chief Specialist

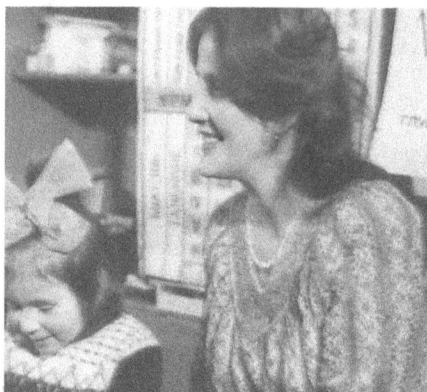

Dr Lyudmila Buteyko (Novozhilova), after the end of her asthma. When she met Dr Buteyko, she had a weight of 120 kilograms and a moustache as a result of active treatment of asthma with steroids. A frame from the film "Dr Buteyko's friends and enemies", Sverdlovsk Film Studio, 1988

Co-author of the Buteyko Method, copyright holder (since 2003), co-founder of the Buteyko Clinic in Moscow (est. 1987), Chief Specialist at the Buteyko Clinic in Moscow (est. 1987).

Lyudmila Buteyko (Novozhilova) met Dr K. Buteyko in 1968, at the age of 31, after twice suffering clinical death as a result of severe attacks of suffocation from bronchial asthma. The emergency doctors spent nights in her house during that time.

Dr K. Buteyko invited her for treatment, and after having assessed her serious condition, told her 9-year-old son Andrey how to reduce her breathing to stop her choking attack and asthma, and the son cured his mother. The choking attacks stopped completely in two weeks, and soon Lyudmila became the most successful Buteyko practitioner and a faithful friend and companion of Dr K. Buteyko for the next 35 years.

Lyudmila was able to transform a difficult medical technology into a simple and accessible form of use, known as the Buteyko Method. Today the Buteyko Method is available to everyone, thanks to Lyudmila Buteyko (Novozhilova).

It is said that Lyudmila can stop a cough or an attack of suffocation in a patient with asthma simply by talking to them on the phone.

Acknowledgements

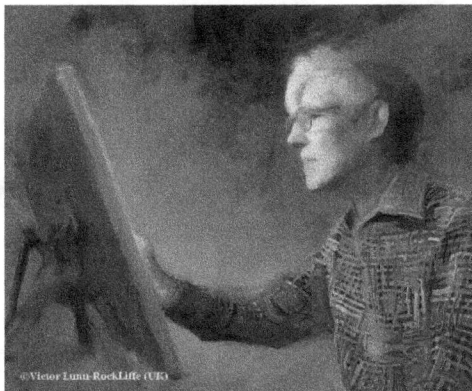

Victor Lunn-Rockliffe, British artist and illustrator, based in London. He was trained in Buteyko breathing in 1997 and was able to completely heal his 25 symptoms within a year.

The authors gratefully acknowledge the contribution made to this book by British artist Victor Lunn-Rockliffe, who has volunteered his work in order to help promote a better understanding of the Buteyko Method.

Special thanks also go to Laura Sophia Scheuerl (Augsburg, Germany), who during the Buteyko classes inspired us to write this book.

In particular the authors would like to thank Dr Andrey E. Novozhilov, co-author of the Buteyko Method and chief physician of the world's oldest Buteyko Clinic in Moscow (est. 1987), for his valuable advice and enthusiastic support in producing this book.

Warning

This book is a guide to the Buteyko breathing exercises

This book is a guide to the most famous part of the Buteyko Method, the Buteyko breathing techniques, but please contact a specialist certified by the Buteyko Clinic in Moscow (est. 1987) to perform the Buteyko breathing exercises, and the Buteyko Method correctly. Check the Specialist's Certificate with its logo, signature of the copyright holder and validity period of one year.

Breathing exercises based on fantasy and non-scientific intervention in breathing can be dangerous

The main difference between the Buteyko breathing techniques and hundreds of old and new breathing exercises is the rigorous scientific approach to breath control.

The rigorous scientific approach to breath control and the key secret of the effectiveness of Buteyko breathing techniques consists in the measurement of breathing. For example, Dr Buteyko for the first time scientifically explains when yoga breathing will help, and when yoga will be deadly.

Just as it is necessary to measure high blood pressure before using medication to control it, it is also necessary to measure breathing to effectively control it.

Breathing is atomic energy; an unreasonable game with breathing leads to insanity and death, warns Dr Buteyko.

Use natural mechanisms of automatic normalization of breathing

Exercises described in this book have a great healing effect if done correctly. As our practice shows, people tend to understand and perform breathing exercises based on volitional, mechanical intervention with breathing: for example, volitional holding of breath after exhalation.

The author Dr Buteyko himself constantly points out that breathing is an automatic process, so the most effective and safe exercises are the ones that automatically normalize breathing without our intervention; for example, exercises of relaxation and correct posture.

Exercises based on volitional intervention in breathing can be dangerous. Exercises based on automatic normalization of breathing are the most effective and safe for everyone.

Dr Novozhilov's explanation of the meaning of the emblem of the Buteyko Method created by Dr Buteyko in 1952

This emblem was created personally by Dr Buteyko many years ago, and it became a registered trademark of the Moscow Buteyko Clinic and the Buteyko Method in 1991.

1. The emblem of the Buteyko Method symbolizes life on Earth. Living matter is built on the basis of chemical compounds of carbon. Carbon is the fundamental element of organic chemistry and of all living things. Each carbon atom links with four others, to form the lattice structure.

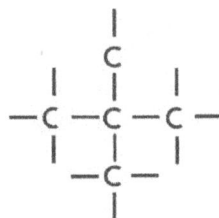

2. The Latin symbol for carbon "C" has been replaced with a circle because the circle is the symbol for perpetual life.

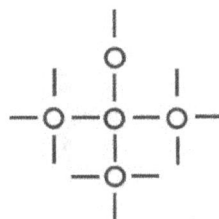

3. The middle carbon atom has been replaced with the globe to signify its central importance to life on Earth.

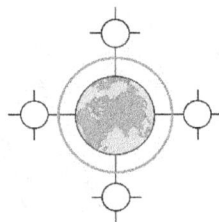

The essence of the Buteyko Method by Dr Andrey E. Novozhilov

Dr Andrey E. Novozhilov, MD

co-author of the Buteyko Method, copyright holder (since 2014)

co-founder and chief physician of the Buteyko Clinic in Moscow (est. 1987)

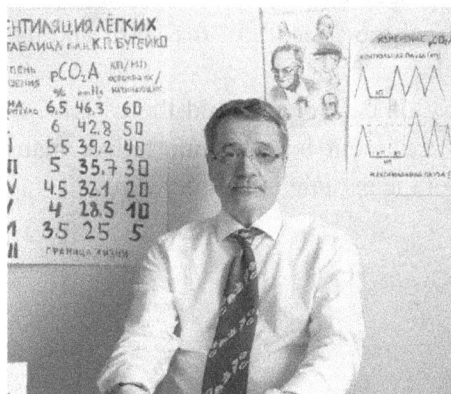

Dr Andrey E. Novozhilov, *chief physician of the Buteyko Clinic in Moscow (est. 1987), 2021*

In this book, the authors talk primarily about the Buteyko breathing technique (BBT) and explain its background.

Nature has given us the ability to control breathing in a wide range, and Dr Buteyko has taught us how to **measure** and **normalize** breathing in order to **maintain and improve health**.

More than half a century ago, the Russian doctor and scientist Dr Konstantin P. Buteyko made a fundamental scientific discovery in medicine and invented a drug-free method of treatment, commonly known as the Buteyko Method.

The Buteyko Method is a complex medical technology, which allows not only the treatment of a number of diseases, but successfully prevents their development in risk groups. Application of only the most popular part of the Buteyko Method, the so-called Buteyko breathing technique (BBT), has saved the lives of millions of people (without any exaggeration) for several generations.

The Buteyko breathing technique has gained the greatest popularity in the treatment of all forms of bronchial asthma, bronchitis, all types of allergies, high blood pressure and high cholesterol, obesity, metabolic diseases and diabetes mellitus, immunity diseases, chronic fatigue, sleep disorders, snoring and sleep apnea. The use of the Buteyko breathing technique protects against frequent colds, from viral infections, allows you to cure a child with enlarged adenoids without surgery to remove them, and much, much more.

According to leading experts in various fields of medical science, Dr Buteyko made a **scientific breakthrough** comparable in importance to the invention of antibiotics or vaccines, that has saved millions of lives. His unique scientific research in the study of respiration allowed Dr Konstantin P. Buteyko to decipher the secret knowledge of Indian yogis about health and Christian ascetics about the strength of the spirit and use this knowledge for the benefit of people.

The idea of the scientific discovery of Dr Buteyko and the essence of the Buteyko Method as a method of treatment is very simple, like many brilliant discoveries and inventions. Let me explain in simple words.

The essence of the Buteyko Method as a design of treatment

As soon as the words about breathing exercises were spoken, it became clear that it would be about the normalization of breathing.

Many people like to say this phrase about the normalization of breathing, but no one explains **what it means and why it is necessary**.

So, the normalization of respiration presupposes the normalization of gas constants in the lungs, in the blood, in cells, at all levels of work of the physiological functional respiratory system. Gas constants are some constant chemical quantities, some constant digits of respiratory gases, of which we have only two in our organism: everyone's favourite oxygen, O_2; and little known by many, carbon dioxide, CO_2. The work of a physiological functional respiratory system is to provide their maintenance within the physiological norm. Oxygen, as we know, we absorb from the air in the process of breathing; whereas carbon dioxide is produced in the cells of the organism in the process of metabolism and is to be removed. Perhaps many will be surprised to learn that the constant of CO_2 is maintained 10 times more accurately than the oxygen constant. This indicates its importance for metabolism and our health.

The laws of the organism's life

The laws of the organism's life are studied through a science called physiology. Our organism is a complex of so-called physiological functional systems, and each of them maintains specific constants within the physiological norm. The coordinated and normal work of all functional systems of the organism ensures what we call our health.

Here are examples of the most important and well-known constants, the maintenance of which within the physiological norm is a prerequisite for our health:

- the organism's temperature is always 36.6 degrees and is a constant value;
- arterial blood pressure is 120/80 mm Hg and is constant;
- blood sugar is always 5 mmol/L and is a mandatory constant for health;
- the oxygen content in the blood is at least 93%, and the carbon dioxide in the lungs is at least 6.5%. These gas parameters are also constant values or constants, the maintenance of which within the physiological norm is strictly monitored by the corresponding functional systems of the organism.

Dozens of key constants or constant values maintain the so-called *homeostasis*, or the constancy of the internal environment of the organism, which as a result determines our health.

Many of these constants are of critical or key importance for maintaining health. Therefore, when they change, powerful compensatory reactions arise from various physiological functional systems, and the work of these compensatory reactions tends to normalize the changed constants.

For example, when the constant of carbon dioxide (CO_2) in the lungs changes, which happens mainly as a result of excessive, deep breathing, we see how in some people the airways get closed and corresponding diseases occur, ranging from chronic rhinitis to bronchial asthma. The severity of the disease is in direct proportion to the change of its specific constant.

Scientific research and discoveries by Dr Buteyko have shown that **a number of diseases arise as a result of the work of compensatory reactions. The essence of these reactions is the normalization of the constants,** homeostasis and, ultimately, the work of the corresponding functional system of the organism.

Dr Buteyko's research has shown that **successful treatment of such diseases should be based on the normalization of specific constants and the normalization of the work of the body's functional system**, which ensures their maintenance.

In this example, both chronic rhinitis and bronchospasm are specific compensatory reactions of the functional system of respiration. These compensatory reactions strive to normalize the CO_2 constant in the lungs, and it is possible to get rid of such diseases only if the respiratory constants and respiratory homeostasis are normalized.

A fundamentally new theory of bronchial asthma by Dr Buteyko

Dr Buteyko created a fundamentally new theory about the appearance of bronchial asthma. He explained the mechanism of this disease, which is based on a change in gas constants and a violation of respiratory homeostasis, and published an article in a scientific medical journal in which he described the key influence of the CO_2 constant on the formation of reversible bronchial obstruction (reversible blockage of the airways).

Today, the scientific medical community believes that the main cause of *reversible bronchial obstruction* and *bronchial asthma* itself is *chronic allergic inflammation of the bronchi*. Clinical manifestations of asthma (coughing, choking attacks, etc.) depend on the activity of *allergic inflammation of the bronchi*. The use of steroids in the treatment of asthma can reduce the activity of *allergic inflammation of the bronchi* and control the course of asthma, but steroids are not able to eliminate *allergic inflammation of the bronchi* completely or get rid of the asthma.

A scientist who discovers how to eliminate *allergic inflammation of the bronchi* forever will effectively answer the question of how to eliminate asthma and will no doubt become a laureate of the Nobel Prize in Medicine and Physiology.

For more than half a century, we have been successfully using *the Buteyko Method* for the treatment of asthma, which clinically proved an undoubted connection between the CO_2 *constant* in the lungs and *allergic inflammation of the bronchi* in patients with bronchial asthma. Clinical practice convincingly demonstrates that normalization of the CO_2 *constant* in the lungs reduces the activity of *allergic inflammation of the bronchi* until its complete elimination. This dependence makes it possible to cure bronchial asthma completely. We have cases of clinical remission of bronchial asthma lasting more than half a century, provided that the CO_2 constant in the lungs is normalized.

For more detail, read the entry on 'CO_2-deficient theory of bronchial asthma by Dr Buteyko' in the Glossary.

A fundamentally new method of treating bronchial asthma by Dr Buteyko

Dr Buteyko invented a fundamentally new method of treating bronchial asthma, based on the normalization of the CO_2 constant, the normalization of the external respiration system, and the normalization of respiratory homeostasis in general.

Scientific research by Dr Buteyko has proven that in patients with bronchial asthma, reversible bronchial obstruction and bronchospasm occur as a result of changes in the CO_2 constant in the lungs and are able to eliminate themselves as soon as respiratory homeostasis and the external respiratory system are being normalized.

Knowledge of this pattern allows the treatment of asthma and related diseases without drugs, provided that the CO_2 constant in the lungs is normalized with the help of the Buteyko breathing technique and dosed physical activity. Dosed physical activity and sports significantly contribute to the normalization of the CO_2 constant. Therefore, with the correct use of physical activity under the control of the increase of ventilation of the lungs, it is possible to successfully normalize the CO_2 constant at all levels of work of the respiratory system and successfully treat asthma or normalize blood pressure without drugs.

The essence of Dr Buteyko's scientific discovery

In other words, the essence of the scientific discovery by Dr Buteyko and the Buteyko Method as a method of treatment is very simple:

- either we normalize gas constants and completely get rid of asthma, allergies, high blood pressure and high cholesterol,
- or else our organism, without taking into account our desire, will strive to normalize respiratory homeostasis with the help of specific and negative compensatory reactions (bronchospasm, vasospasm, high cholesterol and atherosclerosis), and we will fight all our life with diseases that arise as a result of their work.

The Buteyko breathing technique and physical activity (sports) allow you to normalize breathing and completely cure asthma, allergies, normalize blood pressure, cholesterol, normalize sleep, get rid of snoring, chronic fatigue, and stop colds. And all of this - without medication.

Three ways of treatment by the Buteyko Method

Based on the above, the Buteyko Method offers three ways of treatment and recovery.

1. Buteyko breathing techniques or exercises

Buteyko breathing techniques or exercises allow the patient to normalize breathing and respiratory homeostasis to the level of eliminating the symptoms of the disease and reducing drug treatment.

Types of Buteyko breathing exercises

1. Natural methods to eliminate excessive ventilation of the lungs by relaxing and by correcting posture.

2. Volitional methods to eliminate excessive ventilation of the lungs with the help of volitional reduction of breathing depth or volitional breath holding.

3. A combination of natural and volitional ways of breathing normalization.

4. A combination of natural and volitional methods of breathing normalization in combination with dosed physical (muscular) activity under the control of the dynamics of pulmonary ventilation.

(See the entry on 'Buteyko breathing exercises' in the Glossary.)

2. Dosed physical (muscular) activity

Dosed physical (muscular) activity (under the control of the dynamics of pulmonary ventilation) to normalize gas constants and respiratory homeostasis by increasing the activity of metabolism.

Muscle activity allows one to normalize respiratory homeostasis naturally without performing unnatural fictional and always dangerous volitional intervention in the automatic process of the respiratory system.

3. Search, analysis and elimination of the causes of deep breathing

Search, analysis and elimination of the causes of excessive breathing for the prevention of respiratory homeostasis disorders and exacerbation of the disease.

The essence of the Buteyko breathing technique (BBT) by Anna Novozhilova

Anna Novozhilova

Director of the programme 'Genuine Buteyko breathing techniques from Primary Sources for Foreigners'

Certified Buteyko Method specialist of the Buteyko Clinic in Moscow (est. 1987)

"You should feel your breathing and reduce it by one quarter."

Dr Konstantin P. Buteyko, MD, PhD, author of the Buteyko Method

It is impossible to reduce the Buteyko Method as a system of treatment to just breathing exercises. Dr Buteyko always refused to call the Buteyko Method just a complex of breathing exercises. He said that we breathe constantly, day and night, and if the work of the respiratory system is disrupted and diseases have appeared, then for successful treatment it is necessary to normalize the work of the respiratory system, which is functioning constantly, whereas exercises can be done only for a short period of time. Dr Buteyko said that our health requires the respiratory system to work normally all the time, day and night, and not just while doing exercises.

No 'old' or classic Buteyko practitioner who learned from Dr Buteyko himself and then worked for many years as a Buteyko specialist will ever say that the Buteyko Method is just a set of breathing exercises. Any experienced Buteyko practitioner will say that the Buteyko Method is about a healthy lifestyle and a huge complex of knowledge that allows you to normalize the work of the respiratory system in order to maintain and improve your health.

Dr Lyudmila Buteyko, my grandmother, who was Dr Buteyko's wife for over 40 years and worked alongside him all those years as a Buteyko practitioner, used to say that if we do not want to do silly breathing exercises for the rest of our lives, then we must learn to feel and understand our breathing, understand how breathing changes in different situations and be able to normalize the respiratory system in order to prevent illness or successfully treat illness without medication.

Dr Peter Kolb from Australia, who wrote several good short books about the Buteyko Method, said that Dr Lyudmila Buteyko had a rare gift to *tune the breathing, do breathing tuning*' and taught patients to feel their breathing, to 'tune' their breathing and understand how breathing changes. She taught them to normalize breathing in any situation easily, without effort and with pleasure. Lyudmila Buteyko then passed on this rare gift to her students.

The Buteyko breathing technique and the correct measurement of the Control Pause will help you to learn to feel your breathing, and understand how breathing changes in different situations in life. This subtle sensitivity to breathing helps to effectively normalize the respiratory system and successfully treat diseases without medication.

The correct measurement of the Control Pause creates a fine sensitivity to breathing, which allows you to effectively normalize the work of the respiratory system.

The Buteyko breathing technique **forms an understanding of how breathing changes** in different life situations, but the Buteyko breathing technique in most cases does not sufficiently normalize the work of the breathing system, since it is performed only for a limited time.

For successful treatment, preservation and improvement of health, we must ourselves, without the constant implementation of the Buteyko breathing technique, learn to normalize the work of the respiratory system, based on our delicate sensitivity to breathing and our understanding of how breathing changes, then use the various methods to 'fine tune' our breathing.

Professor Buteyko used to say that it is not necessary to learn and use all types of Buteyko exercises (in walking, in jogging, breath holds, mouse etc.); it is enough to do just one exercise to cure asthma, for example. But people are psychologically different and tend to choose the most effective and comfortable exercises for them.

The key idea is that Professor Buteyko hated the word 'exercise'. He used to say: 'My method can be explained in 2 minutes. Otherwise, there's no point explaining it. The whole explanation is about diminishing the depth of breathing, diminishing the inhale. Then there are different exercises in accordance with the psychology of each patient: 70% of people cannot relax and they do not understand it; the remaining 30% dislike sport and they will never do breath holds while walking or jogging.'

One time, I was revising my notes and getting ready for a Buteyko class with Laura and Claudia (Claudia is one of our most successful patients who has achieved a morning Control Pause of 2 minutes, and now she is an experienced Buteyko practitioner in Germany). I decided to consult Dr Andrey Novozhilov, and these were his words: 'Remember that there is no point in learning all types of exercises and doing them. It is better to find the one that is comfortable for you, your favourite one, and learn how to use it till you perfect it. Professor Buteyko always welcomed it if the patient came up with or invented their own exercise which could be checked with two important indicators: whether the symptoms have gone, and whether your CP is growing after doing this exercise. In other words, if you have achieved success and reached a CP of 2 minutes, it means you have already invented your own way/exercise of breathing normalization.'

Buteyko Lessons
by Anna Novozhilova

Director of the programme 'Genuine Buteyko breathing techniques from Primary Sources for Foreigners'

Certified Buteyko Method specialist of the Buteyko Clinic in Moscow (est. 1987)

Class 1. The volitional way to control and normalize the depth of breathing. Control Pause

General terms and understanding

First of all, what is the difference between the Buteyko Method and qigong, yoga and other techniques which involve breathing?

The Buteyko Method is a scientific discovery that essentially is about the MEASUREMENT and NORMALIZATION of respiratory constants and respiratory homeostasis. Breathing is a key function of the human organism, and like every function it can be measured in numbers and figures. And only if there is a deviation from the norm should one start doing breathing exercises in order to normalize the breathing function step by step. The method incorporates a simple, effective system for measuring your state of health.

Normally, we have 5 litres of air per minute going through our lungs (that is in the state of relaxation, normal state). This gives us the necessary quantity of oxygen. However, if this figure of 5 litres/1 minute increases under the same metabolic conditions, hyperventilation of the lungs occurs. This means that the incoming quantity of oxygen at the metabolic level

Changes in the pattern of breathing during pulmonary hyperventilation

one minute

The volume (amount) of air that passes through the lungs, measured in litres per minute

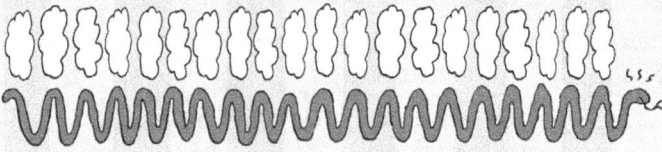

over 15

Pulmonary hyperventilation, severe disease

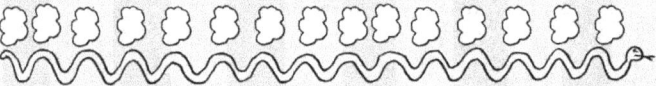

over 10

Pulmonary hyperventilation, moderate to severe course of the disease

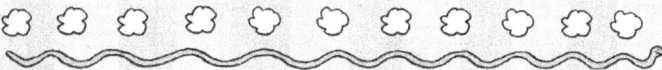

over 5

Deep breathing, the beginning of an exacerbation of the disease

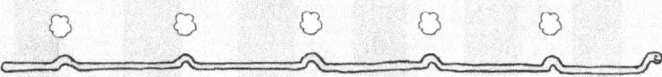

3 - 5

Normal breathing, excellent health

1. Change in breathing pattern during pulmonary hyperventilation

automatically decreases in the same way as excessive breathing increases. IT IS THE LAW OF PHYSIOLOGY.

In other words, the MORE your excessive breathing increases, the LOWER becomes your incoming quantity of oxygen.

Some people are constantly in a hurry and stress a lot, so they never think about their breathing or pay attention to their breathing. When the work of the respiratory system is disrupted, people do not notice this, and diseases arise in response to this, but no one thinks that diseases are associated with the work of the respiratory system. Nobody has ever taught us to pay attention to our breathing. Often breathing is something completely unknown and unclear.

So, let's start with understanding your picture of respiration. Imagine a graphic illustration of the process of respiration, a drawing of respiration:

- Try to feel the process of inhaling and exhaling: what sensations tell you that you have inhaled, and what sensations tell you that you have exhaled.
- Try to feel the movement of air in your nose or in your chest.
- Try to feel the movement of the chest or abdomen during inhalation and exhalation, and tell yourself what sensations of the breathing process are the most vivid.
- Try to draw mentally or imagine a graphic drawing of your breathing and say whether the inhalation is equal to the exhalation or not, what is the breathing rate, is there a cessation of breathing after exhalation or not.

This sensation of your breathing and sensitiveness to your breathing picture will help you later to do breathing exercises.

In the picture the breathing is illustrated as a snake to make it easier to understand.

Devote some time to understanding your breathing and do not be in a hurry to start the exercises. Learn to feel your breathing first.

How to measure
Control Pause correctly

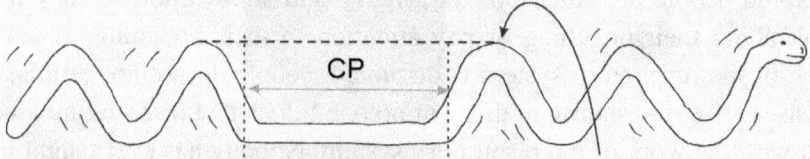

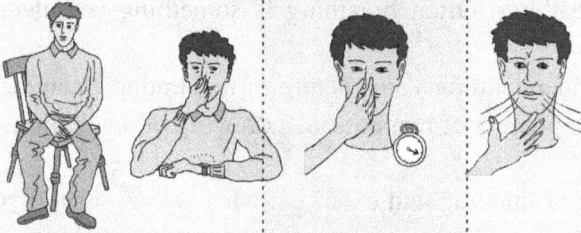

The main feature
of the correct measurement of the Control Pause (CP)
is the presence
of the normal depth of breathing after measurement.

If the depth of the first breath after measuring the CP
is increased, then this is called
the Maximum Pause (MP) or Breath Hold.

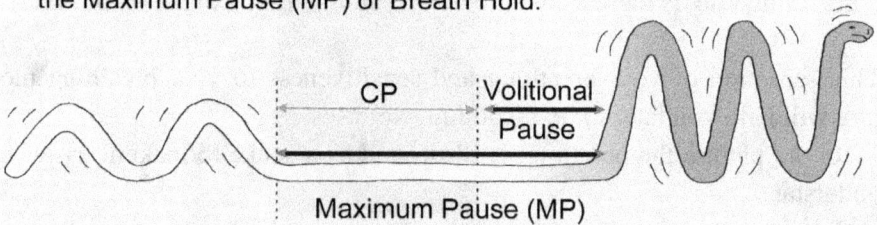

2. How to measure Control Pause correctly

Measuring your CP

'To reduce breathing is some sort of art. Many people are born with the talent to feel their breath and reduce the depth of breathing. This talent, like any other and like any art must be developed and directed in the right way.'

Dr Andrey E. Novozhilov, co-founder and chief physician of the Buteyko Clinic in Moscow (est. 1987)

Always start each Buteyko class by measuring the Control Pause

Correct measurement of the Control Pause develops a fine sensitivity to breathing, develops sensitivity to changes in breathing and helps to perform Buteyko breathing techniques correctly.

Control Pause (CP) is the length of time you can hold your breath without discomfort.

In other words, it implies how long we can stop our breathing (it is measured in seconds) after a normal exhalation without any effort. After the breath hold, your first inhalation should be calm. The entire breath hold must be completely EFFORTLESS. As soon as you feel the first need to breathe again, release your nose and resume breathing. The depth of your first inhalation must be the same as it was before you started holding your breath. The idea is to FEEL the moment when you need to open your nose and breathe in as normally as if you had never held your nose and measured anything. This exercise helps to develop the sensitiveness / delicacy to your breathing that will protect you from hyperventilation in the future.

The most important thing to remember is that the depth of your first breath in at the end of the CP measurement should not be deeper than it was just before you started the breath hold.

In general, one should measure CP in the morning after waking up, without getting out of bed. Just measure it while lying down.

A morning CP of 45 seconds shows us that the CO_2 pressure in the lungs matches the norm. If your CP is less than 45 seconds, it means you have a deficit of CO_2 in the lungs. Of course it is impossible to achieve this

Exercise "Volitional liquidation of deep breathing"

The Art of reducing breathing depth by slight volitional effort

Try to reduce the amplitude of breathing REASONABLY.

REASONABLE – this means reducing the amplitude until you feel a slight hunger for air and by only a quarter or less.

1/4 or less

The key to this exercise is a SLIGHT volitional effort and SLIGHT hunger for air.

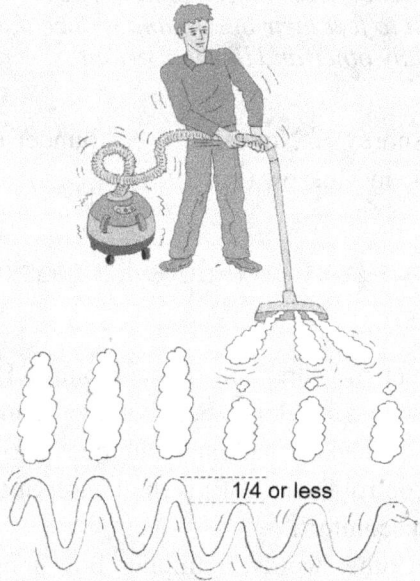

SLIGHT hunger for air DOES NOT CHANGE breathing pattern.

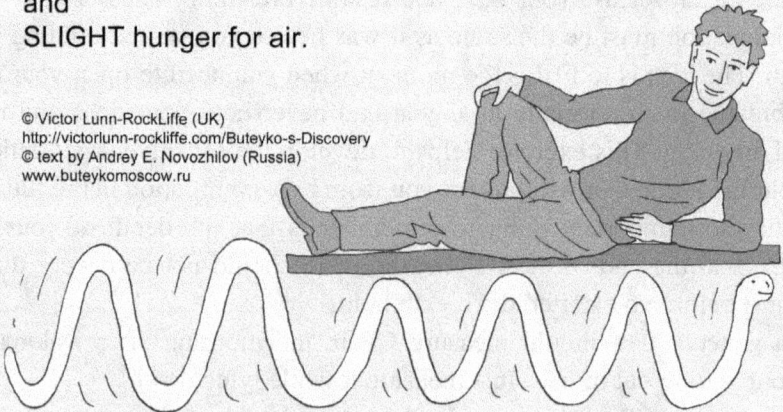

The image of a snake shows a pattern of breathing

3. Exercise: Volitional liquidation of deep breathing

result after one exercise. If you continue to practice the Buteyko Method, gradually your CP will increase to the norm.

Your CP should grow by 5 seconds after each Buteyko session. This shows that you have done everything correctly and practiced long enough.

Exercise 1. 'Volitional liquidation of deep breathing'

The art of reducing the depth of breathing with a light volitional effort or The art of ephemeral, imperceptible breathing

The art of ephemeral, imperceptible breathing is one of the most challenging and interesting exercises

2,500 years ago, the great Chinese philosopher Lao Tzu described the technique of this exercise very accurately: 'A Perfect Man Breathes as if he is not Breathing'.

The name of the exercise reflects the essence of the exercise. The patient should make a decrease in the depth of breathing, reduce the depth of each inhalation, so that a feeling of a slight hunger for air appears.

The main feature of this exercise is a slight decrease in the depth of breathing.

The key to performing the exercise correctly is in the words: slight decrease, gentle decrease, slight and pleasant decrease in breathing

The essence of the exercise 'Volitional liquidation of deep breathing' or the essence of 'The art of elusive, imperceptible breathing' lies in the slight and inconsiderable reduction of the depth or amplitude of breathing, so that the picture of breathing does not change significantly. Look at picture 3.

Exercise "Mouse"

A white cloud is a sick child's deep and noisy breaths.

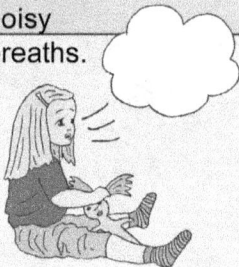

A figurative comparison with the breathing of a little mouse

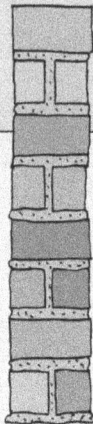

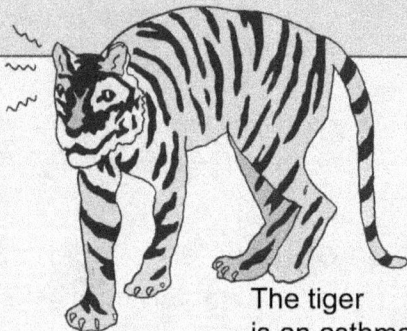

The tiger is an asthma.

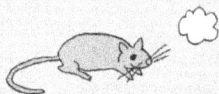

The white cloud shows breathing of a little mouse - shallow, quiet, inaudible, invisible.

The girl tries to breathe shallowly and quietly.

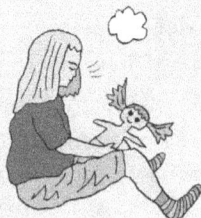

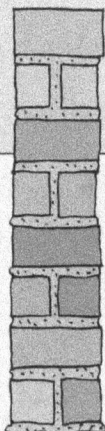

And the asthma goes away because the asthma didn't hear the girl's breathing.

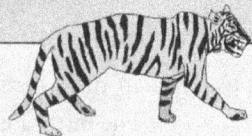

4. A figurative comparison with a little mouse

A figurative comparison with a little mouse's breathing. What is this exercise about?

This exercise also has a figurative comparison with the breathing of a little mouse that hides from an angry, hungry big cat. The mouse's breathing is not audible and not visible. If a hungry cat hears a mouse breathing, he will choose this mouse and eat it. Look at picture 4.

When we have Buteyko classes with children, we explain how a little mouse breathes so that the cunning cat does not hear how the mouse quietly breathes and does not eat it. Asthma behaves in the same way: it chooses and eats someone who has noisy and very noticeable breathing.

Let us imagine this situation: a little mouse needs to cross the path to get home, but suddenly it sees a big cat lying relaxed near its path. The mouse decides to breathe so imperceptibly that the cat does not hear it nor pay attention to it. So it crosses the path unnoticed and gets home successfully.

It works the same way with a child and a disease. For example, if the child breathes loudly, deeply and with an open mouth, some disease like asthma can easily spot this and penetrate through the mouth into the child. To escape this sort of situation, follow the example of the above-mentioned mouse. Close your mouth, breathe calmly and not deeply through the nose. And you will be safe and healthy!

Therefore, the exercise has another name, 'Mouse', and here we are talking about the art of breathing, which is not audible and not visible, like a little mouse.

The key to the correct execution of this exercise is that the process of reducing breathing should be easy and pleasant. So the breathing should be reduced slightly, just as a little mouse holds and hides its breath when the mouse sees an approaching cat.

The Art of reducing breathing depth by slight volitional effort or the Art of ephemeral, imperceptible breathing

The image of the snake demonstrates the maintenance of the original breathing pattern.

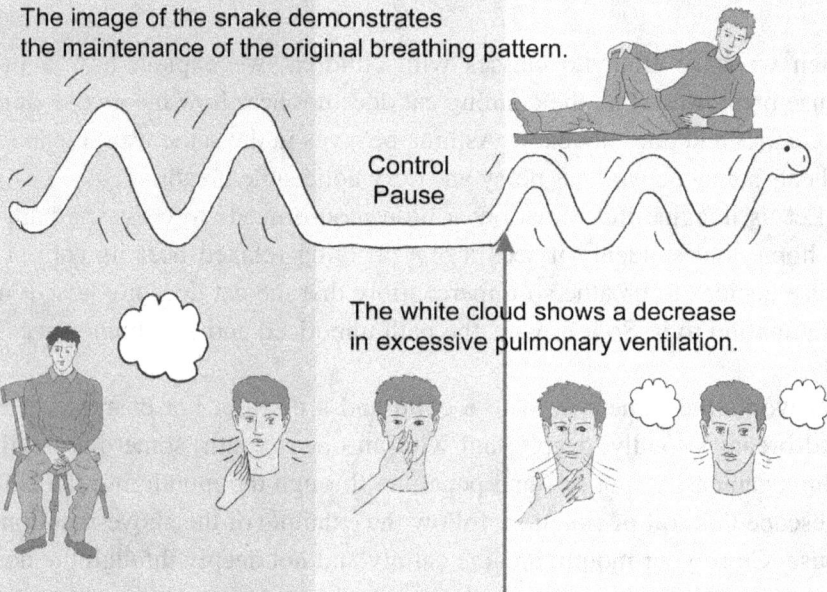

Control Pause

The white cloud shows a decrease in excessive pulmonary ventilation.

Use short and REASONABLE breath holding to get a SLIGHT hunger for air as it happens at the end of the Control Pause.

INTELLIGENT holding of breath brings a SLIGHT hunger for air.

SLIGHT hunger for air DOES NOT CHANGE original breathing pattern.

5. The meaning of 'pleasant air shortage or slight hunger for air'

The techniques of the exercise 'Volitional liquidation of deep breathing' or 'The art of elusive, ephemeral, imperceptible breathing'

After normal exhalation, hold your nose with your fingers and release it at the moment when you feel the first need to breathe. Next, do not breathe in fully. Try to reduce the depth of each inhalation. But this should not cause an increase in your breathing frequency.

In other words, make your first several inhales not as deep as they were. You should feel a small gentle air shortage in your chest.

Continue to reduce the depth of each inhalation, but no more than a quarter or even less, and do it over 1 to 2 minutes; try not to feel any tension in your body.

The air shortage in your chest should be comfortable. There should not be any stress at all.

Remember that the clue to this exercise is gently diminishing the depth of breathing.

The key to the correct execution of this exercise is that the process of reducing breathing should be easy and pleasant. The breathing should be reduced slightly, just as a little mouse holds and hides its breath when the mouse sees an approaching cat.

The main part of the exercise 'Volitional liquidation of deep breathing' is 'a pleasant air shortage or slight hunger for air'. What does this mean?

Air shortage can be described as air hunger.

Your goal is to find a level of pleasant air shortage which allows you to do this exercise for a whole hour without any discomfort. If you reduce the depth of each inhalation too much, then the frequency of your breathing will start increasing. And that is not correct. The effectiveness of the exercise diminishes in this case.

The most important element about this exercise is to CATCH that SLIGHT air shortage. In theory you should reduce it from one tenth to a quarter of your normal amplitude/depth. Of course it is not possible to measure this with a ruler, so you are guided rather by your feelings, sensations. Ask yourself is it comfortable to reduce the depth of my inhalation? Or do I feel any tension and I don't like it?

Don't think at all about your exhalation. Concentrate only on the inhalation. You may also think about measuring your Control Pause. You do not experience any stress and get only the slightest, insignificant air shortage because you release your nose as soon as you feel the first need to breathe. Try to keep this air shortage for 1 to 2 minutes. Reduce only the amplitude, the depth of inhalation. Do NOT interfere with frequency or length of breathing.

Steps of the exercise 'Pleasant air shortage or slight hunger for air'

1. Straighten your back.
2. Do a normal exhalation.
3. Hold your nose with your fingers.
4. With the first need to breathe, release your nose.
5. When you release your nose, try to reduce every inhalation, but not significantly. Reduce it by a small amount so that the air shortage becomes comfortable and the frequency of your breathing does not change. Your inhalation should not be noticeable.

The keyword here is comfortable

Nobody sees what you're doing because only a slight level of concentration is seen on your face. Nothing more, and no struggle.

Now ask yourself: do I feel any tension in my body? Do I like this air shortage? Is it comfortable for me? Is my inhalation noticeable?

Try to keep this slight and comfortable air shortage breathing for 1 to 2 minutes (20 to 30 seconds for beginners), then continue breathing as you wish. Forget about the exercise and think of something else. Then repeat the exercise.

Check yourself

After doing any Buteyko exercise or after each Buteyko class, check yourself with these two questions:

- Does this exercise remove any symptoms I have?
- Is my CP growing by 5 seconds after doing the session of Buteyko exercises?

Class 2. The volitional way to control and normalize the depth of breathing

Always start each Buteyko class by measuring the Control Pause

Correct measurement of the Control Pause develops a fine sensitivity to breathing, develops sensitivity to changes in breathing and helps you perform Buteyko breathing techniques correctly.

First of all, take a look at your breathing: first your breath in, then your breath out. Take your time and look at your breathing.

Now let's measure your CP before starting another Buteyko session. After normal exhalation, stop your breathing and hold your nose with your fingers. The idea is to FEEL the moment when you need to open your nose and breathe in as normally and calmly as if you had not held your nose or measured anything.

When you release your nose, ask yourself if your first breath is equal to the previous one? Or did you suppress it a little? Or is the depth of your first breath increased, but you can easily bring it back to normal with an effort of willpower? Remember that a calm first breath means that the depth of the first breath is not increased and is the same as it was before the CP measurement. Normally, people who have only started to learn Buteyko breathing find it challenging to measure CP, because they try to hold the nose as long as they can, which creates discomfort, while CP measuring implies THE OPPOSITE idea.

How to measure
the Control Pause (CP) correctly

Please remember that there is only one indicator
of the correct CP measurement -
this is the normal depth of the first breath after the measurement.

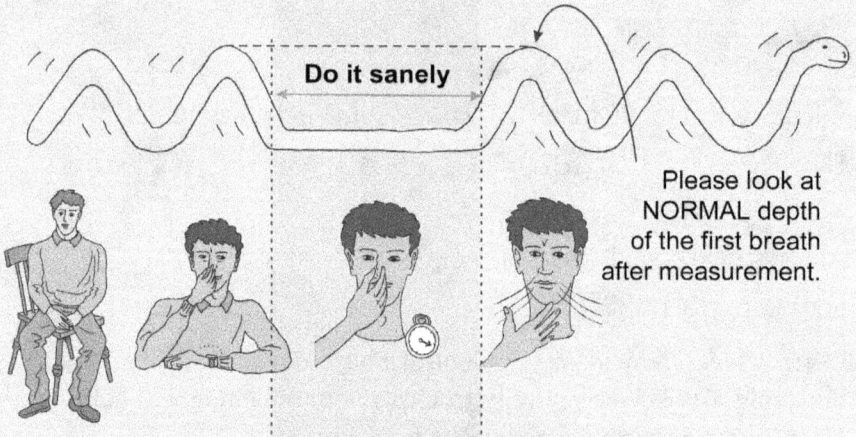

Do it sanely

Please look at
NORMAL depth
of the first breath
after measurement.

For correct CP measurement the duration of holding breath
should be REASONABLE.

REASONABLE - this means to do breath holding without volitional effort.
REASONABLE and without volitional effort - this means to finish breath
holding before the appearance of a slight hunger for air.

The ability to finish holding the breath in good time FORMS the ART
of feeling, understanding and seeing how our breathing is changing.

6. There is one indicator of a correct CP measurement

The goal of each class is to get rid of any symptoms such as blocked nose, cough, mucus, etc. Another goal is to have your CP increased by at least 5 seconds after every session of Buteyko exercises.

Exercise 2. Breath holds after normal exhalation

What is this exercise about?

Start with a correct posture. Do a normal exhalation and hold your nose.

In this exercise you are allowed to bear the air shortage. Do not open your nose with the first wish to inhale. Continue holding your breath and bearing this air shortage REASONABLY. It should be to such an extent that you can control your first few inhalations after opening your nose.

First inhalations should not be deep and noisy.

Try to control the first 3 to 4 inhalations, making them not as deep as you would like. Then come back to normal breathing gradually. The exercise is over and you can breathe as you wish. Take a rest for 30 seconds. Breathe as you'd like to (but not through the mouth!) and think of something else. It is important to forget about breathing for some time to let it become automatic again. Then repeat the exercise.

DURING ANY EXERCISE your face SHOULD NOT demonstrate any struggle with your breathing. In this case the air shortage will be truly pleasant and comfortable. It is a very simple task, but it may become difficult because it is based on your sensitivity.

Exercise 3. Reasonable breath holds + walking

This is a very effective variation on the previous exercise. By adding physical activity, you help your CP grow faster. If you prefer to practise inside, you can just walk around your room.

Things to remember

- Try to keep a correct posture while walking. This automatically helps to diminish the depth of breathing.

Exercise "Reasonable breath holds"

In this exercise, the duration of the volitional breath holding, performed strictly after exhalation, should be REASONABLE and ADEQUATE.

REASONABLE and ADEQUATE duration means that after volitional breath holding it is possible to control the depth of the first 3 to 4 breaths (inhales) and it is possible to calm breathing by holding back (diminishing) its depth during one minute or less.

REASONABLE and ADEQUATE duration means that symptoms of the disease disappear during some minutes.

NOT adequate and NOT reasonable duration of breath holding can provoke increase in the depth of breathing and symptoms of the disease instead of successful treatment.

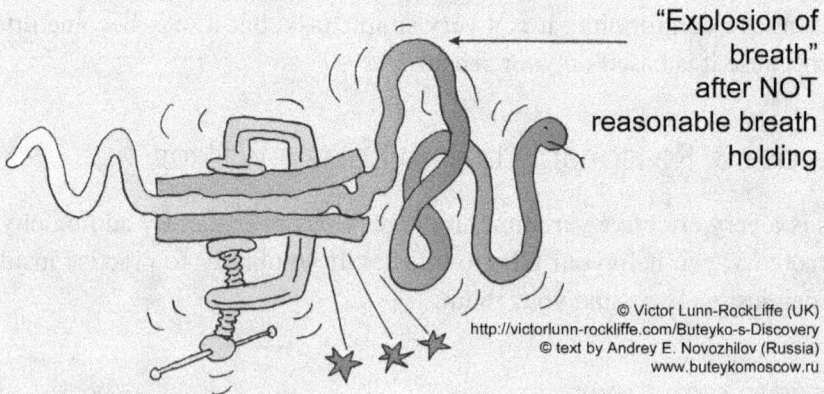

"Explosion of breath" after NOT reasonable breath holding

7. This picture shows the error of not reasonable breath holding and serious air hunger, when one cannot control breathing after releasing the nose

- The air shortage should be reasonable, with no stress or suffering.
- First inhalations are not allowed to be deep and noisy.
- After the exercises, let yourself relax and forget about your breathing for some time.
- The physical activity of walking creates a stronger feeling of air shortage than when you do the exercise while sitting.
- Start with a correct posture.
- Do a normal exhalation, hold your nose and start walking.
- Straighten your back and look straight in front of you.
- Bear a strong air shortage but be REASONABLE. As in sports, it should be reasonable, without any suffering.
- Open your nose and CONTINUE WALKING, trying to keep the air shortage during the first 3 to 4 inhalations by restraining slightly the first 3 to 4 inhalations. First inhalations are not allowed to be deep and noisy. Within the next 15 seconds try to convert the strong air shortage into a mild one. Then maintain this mild air shortage while walking for approximately half a minute.
- Continue walking and *very gradually, step by step* come back to normal breathing.
- Now breathe normally, continue walking and take your time to think of something pleasant. Forget about breathing. Let it become automatic again. Give yourself 1 minute or more to relax. Bend your back if you are tired of the correct posture.

Do not think about your breathing during the break

Nothing should be done to the breathing. Just think about the weather or the ocean. During this minute, the process of breathing becomes automatic again. It is a very important part of the exercise to let the breathing become automatic again.

When one minute's break is over, repeat the exercise.

This exercise should be enjoyable, not stressful. Doing breath holds while walking implies an element of sport: like challenging yourself whether you can do it or not.

Exercise "Reasonable breath holds + walking or slow jogging"

1. After normal breath out hold your nose with your fingers and start walking or jogging. If you choose jogging do it slowly and try to shake a little.

2. While walking or jogging, you need to keep enough strong but REASONABLE and ADEQUATE air shortage.

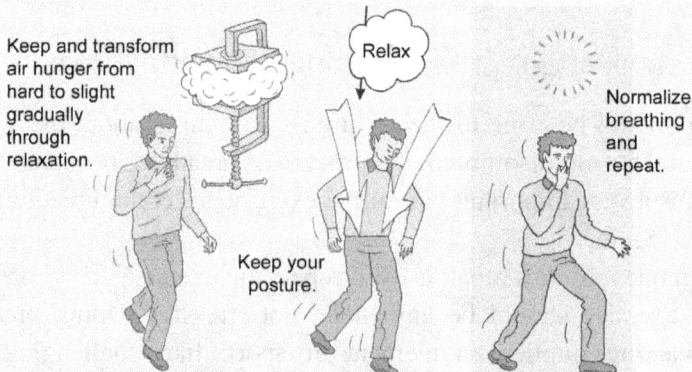

3. REASONABLE and ADEQUATE air hunger means that it is possible to limit the depth of the first few breaths (inhales) and it is possible to control breathing by reducing its depth by volitional effort.

4. After opening your nose keep air shortage and try to transform it from a strong one to a mild one during half a minute, continue walking or slow jogging.

5. Then you continue walking and doing relaxation until your breathing becomes normal, calm and automatic and repeat the exercise.

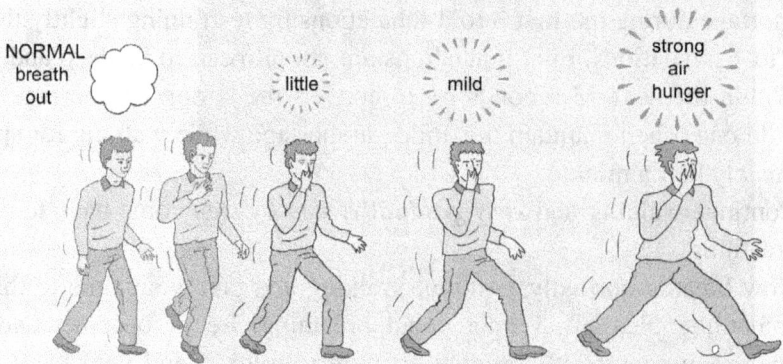

NORMAL breath out   little   mild   strong air hunger

Keep enough strong but REASONABLE and ADEQUATE air shortage.

Keep and transform air hunger from hard to slight gradually through relaxation.

Relax

Normalize breathing and repeat.

Keep your posture.

8. Exercise: Reasonable breath hold while walking or jogging

Exercise 4. Reasonable breath holds + jogging

Combining strong physical activity with the breath hold helps to increase your CP faster. It is good to shake your body while jogging. Add shaking as if you are jumping a bit. If we add jogging to the breath hold exercises, it is important to know that:

- Air shortage will be even stronger, and it will appear to be more difficult to convert it to a mild one.
- Keeping correct posture during jogging will help to diminish the depth of breathing automatically.
- Continue jogging when you release your nose.
- Then proceed to walking only when your air shortage becomes milder and come back to normal breathing in walking.
- Hold your nose and start jogging. It is not about running fast here, more about shaking your body. Try to shake it. At the same time relax everything inside, keeping a small air shortage in your chest, for about half a minute.
- Bear a significant air shortage but be reasonable, do not go to extremes.
- While jogging, you need to try to keep the air shortage, transforming it from a strong one to a mild one during half a minute.
- Then you continue walking and doing relaxation as you wish until your breathing becomes normal and automatic. After 1 minute or more, repeat the exercise.

Exercise "A natural way to control and normalize the depth of breathing"

There are three natural ways to normalize breathing:
- Good posture
- Relaxation
- Reasonable muscle work (sport exercise)

1. Constant hypertonicity of some muscle groups makes us breathe deeply.

2. Poor posture increases the so-called breathing resistance, which forces us to breathe deeply.

3. Hypodynamia inhibits metabolism and disrupts respiratory homeostasis.

So sometimes it is enough to adopt the correct posture and relax to stop a cough, choking attack or normalize blood pressure without medication.

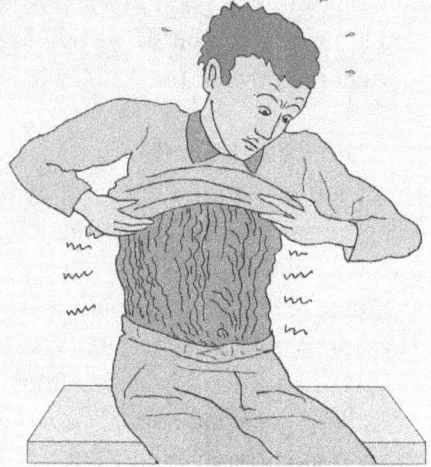

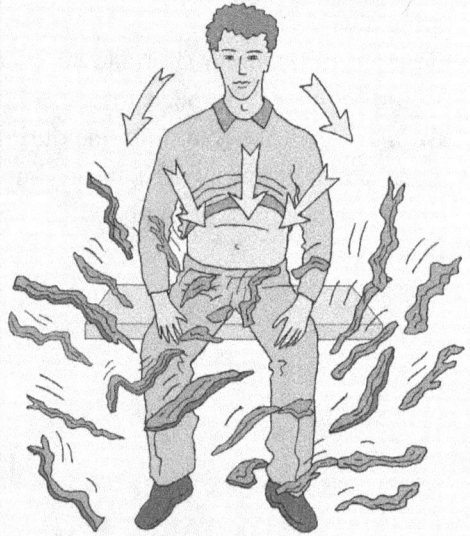

9. Good posture and relaxation skills are a natural way of treatment

Class 3. A natural way to control and normalize the depth of breathing

Always start each Buteyko class by measuring the Control Pause

Correct measurement of the Control Pause develops a good sensitivity to breathing and to changes in breathing, and helps you perform Buteyko breathing techniques correctly.

Exercise 5. Correct posture. Reducing the depth of breathing automatically as a result of correct posture

To start the class, look at your breathing. Notice your inhalation, then your exhalation. Take your time and look at your breathing. Then measure your CP.

Take a look at the people around you. How many of them have their back straight and their shoulders down in a relaxed way? Sadly, the majority of people suffer from a round back and stooped posture. And incorrect posture is one of the main causes of disfunction of the respiratory system.

To get a correct posture, do the following in sequence:

- Stand by a wall, ideally one without a skirting board.
- Gently press the back of your head to the wall.
- Then press your shoulders to the wall by slightly moving them back. Pull your shoulders apart correctly: they should be moved back to the wall and not lifted up.
- Press your tailbone to the wall.
- Press your heels to the wall.

After this, ask yourself whether you feel that your diaphragm has lifted as a result of the good posture? Then take a look at your breathing.

As soon as you feel that your diaphragm or upper abdomen, where the costal arch passes, has risen up or slightly pulled up, your depth of

Exercise "Correct posture is the first natural way to automatically normalize breathing"

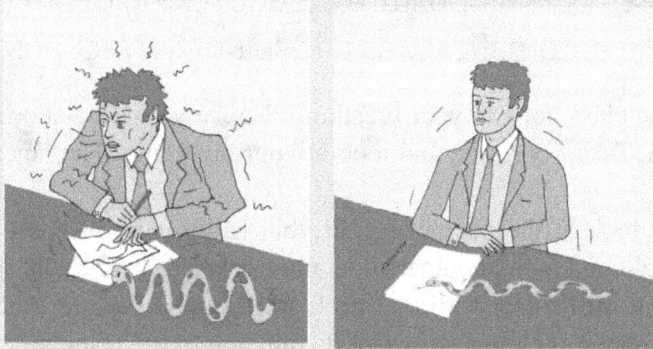

The image of a snake shows how the depth of breathing changes depending on our posture.

Moving shoulders back raises/pulls up/lifts up the diaphragm and the depth of breathing begins to decrease automatically.

The diaphragm or upper abdomen lifted up is the only sign of good posture.

10. Correct posture is crucial

breathing will automatically begin to decrease. This happens as soon as you pull your shoulders back a little and press them against the wall.

If all this is done gently and correctly, you will feel your depth of breathing starts to be reduced automatically as a result of your correct posture.

It may seem that correct posture can build up tension because it feels a bit strange, but here you should concentrate on your inner relaxation.

Always remember two points about correct posture and check yourself: **as soon as your diaphragm is lifted up, the depth of breathing gets reduced automatically.** To do this, you need to straighten your back and pull your shoulders back slightly. This will already start the healing process, the treatment. At this point the respiratory function starts being normalized, and the gas constants in the lungs gradually get normalized too.

An interesting fact
How powerful this exercise is we learned once from a patient who used to suffer from asthma. He told us that he managed to cure it and get rid of the symptoms completely through doing this Correct Posture exercise. He dedicated plenty of time to it and eventually treated his asthma successfully just by standing many hours by the wall with correct posture.

Exercise 6. Relaxation. Reducing the depth of breathing automatically as a result of relaxation

We do nothing with breathing while doing relaxation exercise

In this exercise we do not touch our breathing. We just try to relax the parts of the body which can influence our breathing. For example, arm and legs have nothing to do with the process of breathing, so we do not use them in this exercise.

Do not manipulate your breathing. Just breathe normally, absolutely like you want to breathe. All necessary changes to your breathing will happen **automatically**.

Exercise "Reducing the depth of breathing through sequential relaxation"

The essence of the exercise is in the consistent relaxation of the muscles, the hypertonicity of which force us to breathe deeply.

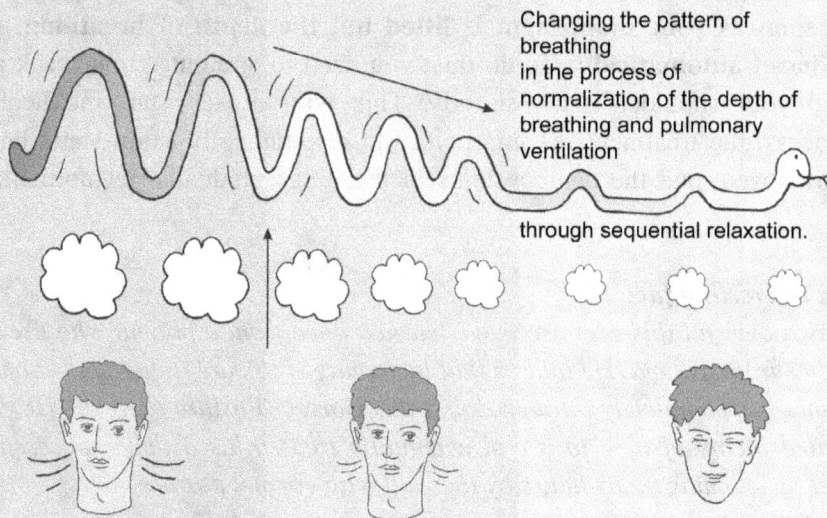

Changing the pattern of breathing
in the process of normalization of the depth of breathing and pulmonary ventilation

through sequential relaxation.

For example, focusing on relaxing facial muscles causes breathing to stop for a short time.
After that, relaxation of the muscles around the eyes reduces the amplitude (depth) of breathing automatically.

Consistent relaxation of other muscles will make breathing not visible and not audible, and the cough will stop, and blood pressure will normalize without medication.

11. Relaxation is the second way to achieve breathing normalization naturally

The first part of relaxation which influences our breathing is our mimic and facial expression. There are three main points here:

Forehead. Imagine that your imaginary wrinkles are straightening, flattening out and your forehead gets rid of them. Do not touch your forehead with your hands, it should all happen mentally.

Muscles around the eyes. Their form is round and we can imagine that they are like glasses. They start growing and relaxing at the same time and you stop blinking because of that, because they are relaxing.

Lower part of the jaw. It should relax and hang down as if opened, but your mouth should still be closed. The face becomes a sort of mask, without emotions.

An interesting fact
A yogi can stare at one point for a whole hour without blinking. The way they do it is to relax the muscles around their eyes.

Back of your head. There is a triangular muscle here; imagine that it is being relaxed while opening up, like a peacock's tail.

Neck and down to your **shoulders**. Imagine a stack of small boxes/bricks (like in children's toys) on your shoulders which are being destroyed. Your shoulders are like those bricks, and they feel relaxed as they move down. It is all fantasy, just a mental image. But don't forget about correct posture now. Straighten your back.

Muscles between the ribs. Imagine that they are relaxing and the ribs draw apart a little. Again, it is just a fantasy.

Upper abdomen from navel to costal arch, upper part of the stomach. Mentally tell this zone to relax inside. But still keep the correct posture and back straight.

The idea is that your breathing becomes automatically reduced when you do all these points of relaxation. It usually takes approximately 40 seconds to relax all these zones.

In this exercise we DO NOT TOUCH THE BREATHING at all.

To the exercises
"Natural ways to automatically reduce the depth of breathing"

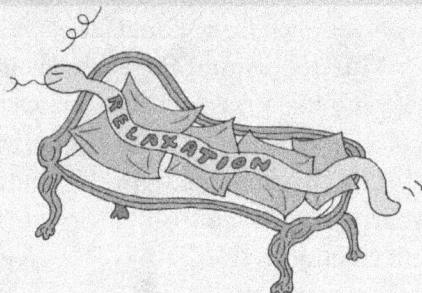

Please note that step-by-step relaxation reduces the depth of breathing AUTOMATICALLY and without hunger for air.

Please note that correct posture reduces the depth of breathing AUTOMATICALLY and without hunger for air.

Moving shoulders apart tightens or slightly moves the diaphragm up and the depth of breathing automatically decreases.

Please note that in these exercises we do not touch the breath.

The depth of breathing decreases AUTOMATICALLY without hunger for air.

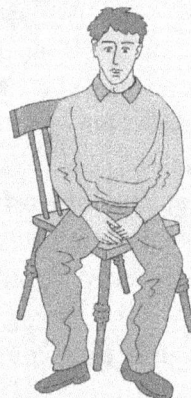

12. To the exercises 'Natural ways to automatically reduce the depth of breathing'

Just check if there is any automatic feedback from the breathing. Is it reduced a bit as a result of relaxation? Concentrate only on relaxation. As a result of this relaxation, you will feel eventually that your depth of breathing becomes automatically reduced.

In general, you should achieve the automatic breath suspension in every point of this relaxation exercise. You relax your forehead, all the wrinkles and you feel that you are not breathing in this moment; you relax the muscles around your eyes and you understand that in this moment you are not breathing. Not on purpose, but automatically, as a result of this relaxation. That's the phenomenon of concentration, your attention on some point. Concentration of your attention on some point always stops the breathing automatically.

You move from one point of relaxation to another, not thinking about inhales or exhales. It is just in each point that the breathing is stopped for a moment or a few seconds.

During relaxation, the air shortage or slight hunger for air will not appear

This is the phenomenon of this exercise: the depth of breathing clearly gets reduced, but **an air shortage does not appear**. Only from the general sensations of breathing you do understand that your breathing has significantly and undoubtedly reduced. This is the reason why Dr Buteyko classified this exercise as **a natural way to control breathing**, in contrast to all other exercises in which we intervene directly with breathing.

During relaxation the air shortage must not appear, otherwise there will appear tension at the same time, which you will use for keeping and maintaining the air shortage. And if the tension is strong enough, the process of relaxation will stop - that makes the combination of the exercises really hard: you do the relaxation, but if the air shortage appears as a result of breathing getting reduced, this air shortage should be very insignificant in order to be able to keep doing relaxation.

Exercise "How to breathe during a long conversation or speech without deep breathing"

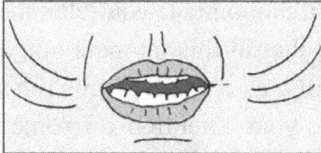

To prevent deep breathing during a long conversation, you must follow two simple rules:

- you can only inhale through your nose,

- your inhale should be almost imperceptible.

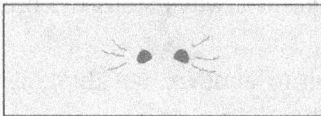

How can you breathe through your nose during a long conversation?

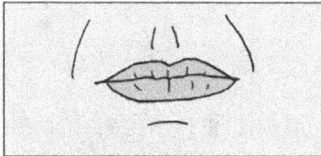

These rules can be followed while reading any text aloud.

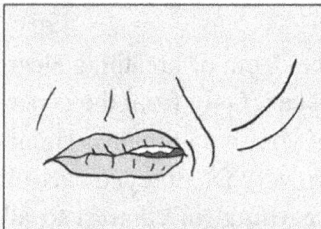

Demonstrative breathing through the mouth during a conversation psychologically always plays against the speaker, and in asthmatics or hypertensive patients it provokes coughing, suffocation, increased blood pressure and other troubles.

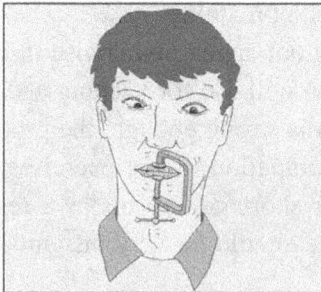

13. How to breathe during a long conversation

Exercise 7. How to breathe during a long conversation or speech without deep breathing

The purpose of the exercise is to learn **how to inhale through the nose**, and not through the mouth, **during a long conversation or speech.**
Inhalation through the mouth during conversation always leads to hyperventilation of the lungs and an attack of bronchial obstruction or other symptoms.

To learn how to inhale only through the nose during a long conversation, try reading a text aloud. Take any book and read aloud, following **two rules**:

- you can only inhale through your nose,
- the **inhalation** should be almost **imperceptible**.

Normally we all speak as we exhale. We cannot speak while breathing in or when breathing stops. Our voice appears and sounds only during the exhalation. However, at the end of an exhalation, the air in the lungs ends and we must inhale. This is the most common and natural process. It is at this very moment that you need to close your mouth and **inhale through your nose**, after which you can continue to speak, making a natural exhalation.

After a while, the air in your lungs will run out again and you will want to take a breath in. At this point, you need to close your mouth and breathe in through your nose, after which you can continue reading aloud or talking.

The second requirement in this exercise is to try to inhale through your nose very quietly, without demonstration, imperceptibly. To achieve this, it is necessary to interrupt your speech on time and not squeeze all the air out of your lungs. Close your mouth and take a quiet and imperceptible breath in through your nose. Again, we are talking about catching that right moment to close your mouth and make a quiet inhalation, before you run out of breath completely. To do this, you need to monitor the rhythm and speed of your speech. If the speech is very fast and you want to say a lot at once, then the inhalation will always occur through the mouth and result in hyperventilation and consequent symptoms.

How to measure
Control Pause (CP) correctly?

Please remember that the depth of the first breath
after the measurement should be normal.
This is the main sign of correct measurement.

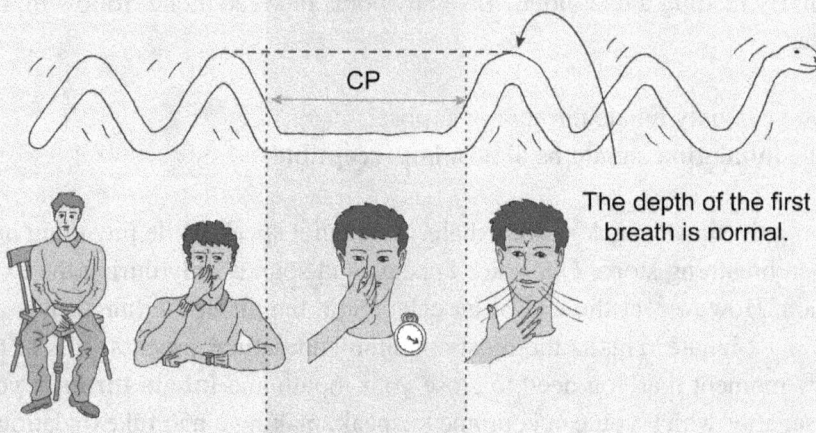

CP

The depth of the first
breath is normal.

The image of the snake shows that the depth of breathing
did not increase after measuring CP.

The duration of the volitional holding of breath
should be REASONABLE.

REASONABLE - this means that the depth of breathing has
not increased after measuring CP.

14. The main sign of the correct measurement of CP

By doing this exercise, you will very quickly find your personal tempo and rhythm of speech, observing how you can quietly and imperceptibly breathe in through your nose, which is 100% protection against the appearance of negative symptoms after a long conversation or communication.

Class 4. Combinations of the Buteyko breathing techniques without physical activity to increase treatment effect

Always start each Buteyko class by measuring the Control Pause

Correct measurement of the Control Pause develops a fine sensitivity to breathing, develops sensitivity to changes in breathing and helps you perform Buteyko breathing techniques correctly.

At the end of every class, take your time to relax and let your breathing become automatic; then measure your CP again. If it is augmented by 5 seconds, this is an indicator that you have been doing everything correctly and have practised enough times.

Combination 1. Correct posture + Relaxation

Stand by the wall and do the correct posture exercise. Straighten your back, pull your shoulders apart slightly, see if your diaphragm is lifted up automatically (as a result of your shoulders being pulled apart) and the depth of your breathing reduced too.

Now add relaxation.

Follow all the steps and spend no more than 40 seconds doing it.

Forehead. Imagine that the imaginary wrinkles are straightening, flattening out and the forehead gets rid of them. Do not touch the forehead with your hands, it should all happen mentally.

Muscles around the eyes. Their form is round and we can imagine that they are like glasses. They start growing and relaxing at the same time and

Exercise "Combination 1. Correct posture + Relaxation"

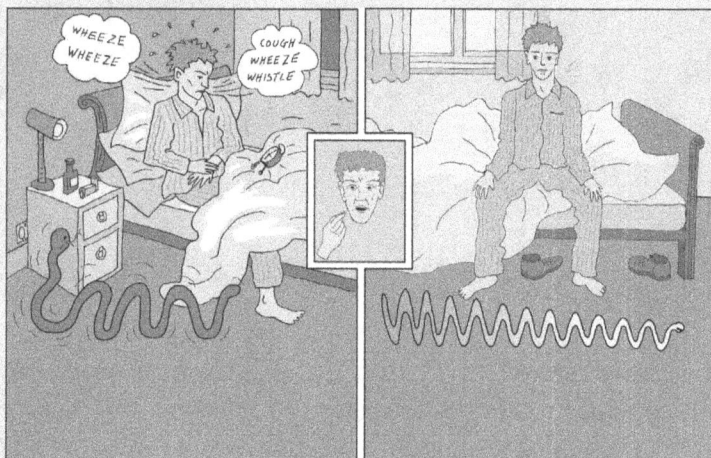

If you are trying to stop the onset of an attack with a combination of correct posture and relaxation, then always start with the correct posture, which reduces the depth of breathing AUTOMATICALLY and does NOT require intervention in breathing.

Buteyko exercises that reduce the depth of breathing automatically and indirectly
are always safe and as effective as possible.

15. Combination 1

you stop blinking because of that, because they are relaxing.

Lower part of the jaw. It should relax and hang down as if opened, but your mouth should still be closed.

Back of your head. There is a triangular muscle here; imagine that it is relaxing while opening up, like a peacock's tail.

Neck and down to the shoulders. Imagine a stack of small boxes/bricks (like children's toys) on your shoulders which are being destroyed. Your shoulders are like those bricks, and they feel relaxed as they move down. It is all a fantasy, you are doing it mentally. Don't forget about correct posture. Straighten your back.

Muscles between the ribs. Imagine that they are relaxing and the ribs drawing apart a bit. Again, it is all fantasy.

Upper part of the stomach. Mentally, tell this zone to relax inside. But still keep the correct posture and the back straight.

Now ask yourself whether you feel more relaxed and your breathing is diminished a little as a result of relaxation?

Combination 2. Correct posture + Relaxation + Volitional liquidation of deep breathing ('A mouse', a figurative comparison with a little mouse's breathing near a hungry cat)

Start with the correct posture exercise standing by the wall. Straighten your back, pull the shoulders apart slightly, press the back of your head and heels to the wall. Now try to feel if your diaphragm is lifted up automatically (as a result of your shoulders being pulled apart) and the depth of your breathing reduced too.

Now add relaxation. Follow all the steps and spend no more than 40 seconds on it. Ask yourself whether you feel more relaxed and your breathing is diminished a little as a result of relaxation? If this happens, then make a natural breath out and hold your nose with your fingers. Start the 'Mouse breath' exercise.

With the first need to breathe, release your nose. When you release your nose, try to reduce every inhalation but not significantly. Reduce it a very

Exercise "Combination 2.
Correct posture + Relaxation + 'a Mouse' "

The snake drawing shows the change in the depth of breathing
while MAINTAINING the ORIGINAL breathing pattern.

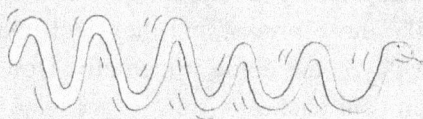

**The keyword here
is comfortable.**

**1. The exercise is performed CORRECTLY.
The exercise has maximum effectiveness.**

The light and comfortable slight hunger for air
that resulted from the third part of the exercise (a mouse)
did not make significant changes in the breathing pattern.

The snake drawing shows that a significant decrease in the depth
of breathing leads to a CHANGE in the ORIGINAL breathing pattern.

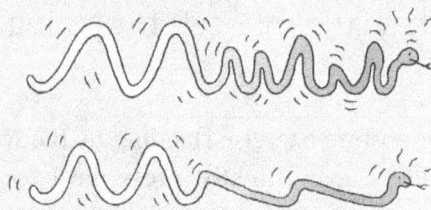

**2. The exercise is performed INCORRECTLY.
The exercise creates discomfort and
has minimal effectiveness.**

The third part of the exercise (a mouse)
made significant changes in the breathing pattern.
Breathing depth is reduced by more than one quarter.

16. Combination 2

little, so that the air shortage becomes comfortable and the frequency of your breathing does not change. Your inhalation should not be noticeable.

The keyword here is comfortable

Nobody sees what you're doing, because only a slight level of concentration is seen on your face. Nothing more and no struggle.

Now ask yourself: Do I feel any tension in my body? Do I like this air shortage? Is it comfortable for me? Is my inhalation noticeable?

Try to keep this slight and comfortable air shortage for 20 to 30 seconds, and then start breathing as you wish. Forget about the exercise and think of something else. Then repeat the exercise.

Combination 3. Correct posture + Relaxation + Reasonable breath hold + Relaxation

Now let's proceed to another combination.

Sit down and straighten your back. Move the shoulders back a little to help your diaphragm lift. It will make the depth of your breathing reduce automatically. Feel your breath, and take your time to see how your breathing behaves.

Now add the Relaxation exercise. Keep your back straight, and start relaxing your forehead, the muscles around your eyes; slacken your jaw and relax the back of your head. Then proceed to other points of relaxation: relax your neck, shoulders, move apart the muscles between your ribs and relax the upper part of your stomach. Continue doing this with your back straight. Repeat the relaxation if needed. You may find it difficult to relax these parts of the body, but with practice it will come.

If you feel that your breathing has reduced as a result of the relaxation, now proceed to the next part of the exercise. After a natural exhalation, hold your nose. When you feel the need to breathe, bear it for some seconds and then release your nose.

Do not let your first inhalations be deep.

Try to convert your strong air shortage into a mild one with the help of relaxation. In other words, try to relax all the above-mentioned parts of

Exercise "Combination 3.
Correct posture + Relaxation
+ Reasonable breath hold + Relaxation"

The effectiveness of the exercise depends on the correct execution of the third part "Reasonable duration of breath holding".

The duration of holding the breath is reasonable, because the depth of the first breath is NORMAL and the breathing pattern has no significant changes.

The exercise has maximum effectiveness.

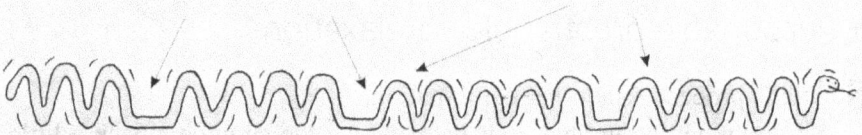

The duration of holding the breath is NOT reasonable, because the depth of the first breath is INCREASED and the breathing pattern has significant changes.

The exercise produces discomfort and has minimal effectiveness.

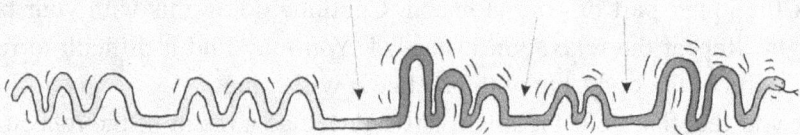

17. Combination 3

your body while converting the air shortage into a mild one. Relaxation is supposed to help make it mild much faster. Continue restraining your first several inhalations, converting the air shortage into a mild one, and then gradually come back to normal breathing.

Take your time, think of something else and breathe normally, as you wish, but only through the nose. Here comes the important part of giving time to your breathing to come back to automatic functioning.

Some patients ask if it is allowed to listen to music during the exercises or watch TV. Usually this means they are not giving the required attention to the exercises. They don't focus enough or don't understand the exercises and eventually they feel bored. In the beginning every part of the exercise requires high attention, so it is not recommended to combine it with watching TV or playing music.

Class 5. Combinations of the Buteyko breathing techniques with physical activity to increase treatment effect

Always start each Buteyko class by measuring the Control Pause

Correct measurement of the Control Pause develops a fine sensitivity to breathing, develops sensitivity to changes in breathing and helps to perform Buteyko breathing techniques correctly.

Remember that the entire breath hold must be completely EFFORT-LESS. As soon as you feel the first need to breathe again, release your nose and resume breathing. The depth of your first inhalation must be the same as it was before you started holding your breath. The idea is to FEEL the moment when you need to open your nose and breathe in as normally as if you hadn't held your nose or measured anything.

Exercise "Combination 4.
Correct posture + Relaxation + Reasonable
breath hold + Walking + Relaxation"

The key to this exercise:
- The effectiveness of this exercise depends on your art of consistent relaxation (lesson "Natural ways to normalize the depth of breathing").
- The ability to perform relaxation controls the reasonableness or the necessary duration of volitional holding of breathing.
- Strong and uncomfortable "hunger for air" will not allow relaxation.
- The ability to perform relaxation sets a reasonable speed of walking.

The duration of volitional breath holding is NORMAL.

The duration of volitional breath holding is clearly EXCESSIVE.

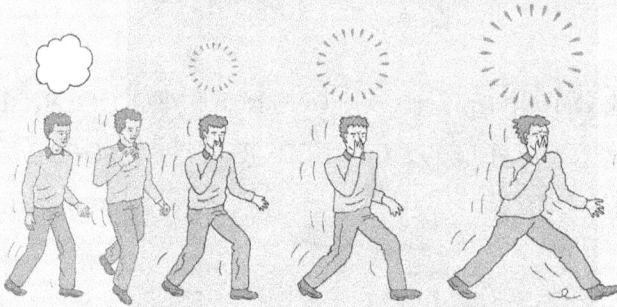

1. Correct posture and start relaxing while walking.

2. Keep reasonable duration of volitional breath holding.

3. Be able to limit the depth of the first few breaths (inhales).

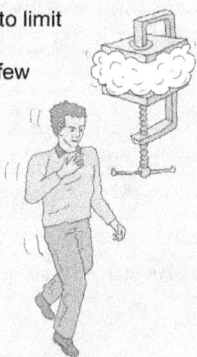

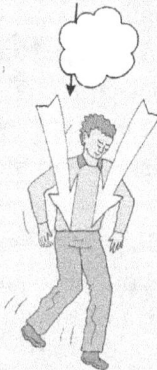

4. Normalize your posture and start relaxing during the first breaths while continuing walking.

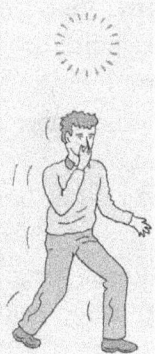

18. Combination 4

Combination 4. Correct posture + Relaxation + Reasonable breath hold + Walking + Relaxation

This combination implies adding physical activity.

Stand by the wall to practise correct posture (back of your head, shoulders, tailbone and heels pressed to the wall) and start doing the Relaxation exercise.

Follow all the steps of Relaxation and spend no more than 20 seconds on it. Ask yourself whether you feel more relaxed and whether your breathing is diminished a little as a result of relaxation? If this happens, then make a natural breath out, hold your nose with your fingers and start walking.

Keep your back straight, look in front of you and continue walking. Bear a strong air shortage but be REASONABLE. Try to add relaxation now while walking and continue bearing the air shortage.

Open your nose and CONTINUE WALKING, converting the strong (but reasonable) air shortage into a mild one during 15 to 30 seconds. First inhalations should not be deep and noisy! At the same time integrate your relaxation, while you convert the strong air shortage into a mild one. Relax all the points (forehead, muscles around the eyes, jaw, back of your head, neck, shoulders, between the ribs and upper part of the stomach) while walking for 1 minute. Relaxing all these parts will help you to achieve the mild air shortage faster. Then maintain it a little more while walking, continuing doing relaxation. Here it means that you are adding the 'Mouse breath' exercise – breathing calmly and imperceptibly as a mouse. Then very gradually, step by step, come back to normal breathing.

Now breathe normally, continue walking and take your time to think of something pleasant. Forget about breathing. Let it become automatic again. Give yourself 1 minute or more time to relax. Bend your back if you are tired of the correct posture, but continue walking and relaxing slightly.

DURING ANY EXERCISE your face SHOULD NOT demonstrate any struggle with your breathing. In this case your air shortage will be truly pleasant and comfortable. It is a very simple task, but it may become difficult because it is based on your sensitivity.

When you are ready, repeat the exercise.

Combination 5. Correct posture + Relaxation + Reasonable breath hold + Jogging + 'The Mouse' + Relaxation

The combination in this class almost repeats those from the previous combination, but with one exception: we add jogging rather than walking. I think it's necessary to clarify what jogging is:

Jogging refers to a light and moderate form of running. Its pace is between walking and running. Jogging implies more shaking your body than when running at a quick pace. This type of jogging is useful as by itself it leads to breathing reduction.

Stand by the wall to practise the correct posture and start doing the Relaxation exercise.

Follow all the steps of Relaxation and spend no more than 20 seconds on it. Ask yourself whether you feel more relaxed and whether your breathing has diminished a little as a result of the relaxation? If this happens, then make a natural breath out, hold your nose with your fingers and start jogging. Remember that it is not about being fast here, rather about shaking your body a little while jogging.

Still try to keep your back straight while jogging; look in front of you and continue jogging. Bear a strong air shortage, but be REASONABLE. Try to add relaxation now while jogging and continue bearing the air shortage. Relaxation while jogging will turn the severe lack of air into a very light one, and the Mouse breathing exercise while jogging will begin.

In case of jogging, the air shortage will be stronger than in walking, because jogging is a stronger physical activity.

Open your nose and CONTINUE JOGGING, converting this strong and hard air shortage into a mild one for 1 minute. First inhalations should not be deep and noisy. At the same time integrate the relaxation, while you convert the air shortage into a mild one. Relax all the points (forehead, muscles around the eyes, jaw, back of your head, neck, shoulders, between the ribs and upper part of the stomach). Relaxing all these parts will help you to achieve the mild air shortage faster. Then maintain it a bit more while jogging, continuing doing the relaxation. Then very gradually, step by step, come back to normal breathing and START WALKING.

Now breathe normally, continue walking and take your time to think of something pleasant. Forget about breathing. Let it become automatic again. Give yourself some minutes or more time to relax and continue walking. Bend your back if you are tired of the correct posture. When you are ready, come back to the wall to practise good posture and repeat the exercise. At the end of the class, do not forget to measure your CP.

Usually, this combination takes some effort because of its strong physical activity and strong air shortage.

How to build Buteyko sessions

It is recommended to do 1 hour of Buteyko exercises in the morning and 1 hour in the evening. 2 hours per day are enough to make your CP grow by 5 seconds gradually if you do everything correctly. Sometimes our patients wonder what is the best way to build the 1 hour Buteyko session? In general, you can do the exercises in any order you like. It is not necessary to do ALL TYPES of the above exercises. Just choose the ones you like and do best, and practise those.

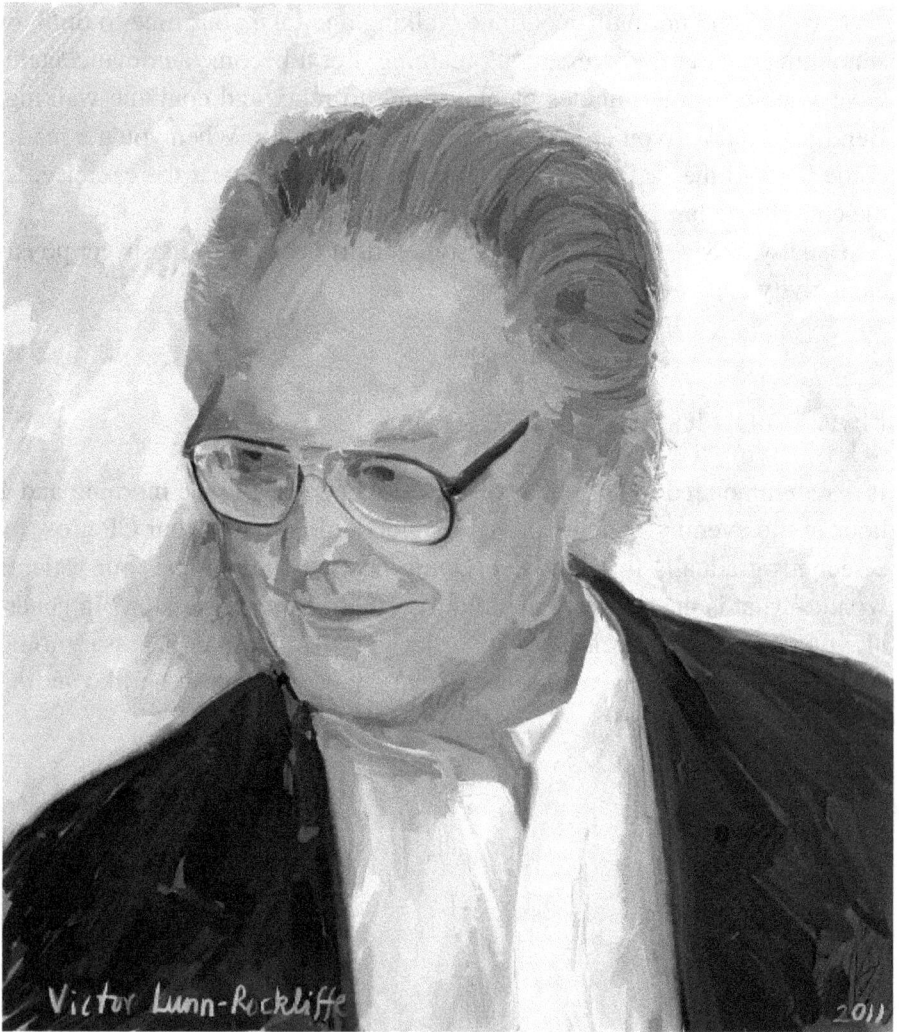

Dr Konstantin P. Buteyko, New Zealand, 2000

Konstantin P. Buteyko, remarkable scientist and brilliant doctor, from the archive, by Dr Lyudmila D. Buteyko (Novozhilova)

co-author of the Buteyko Method, copyright holder (since 2003)

co-founder and chief specialist of the Buteyko Clinic in Moscow (est. 1987)

About Konstantin Buteyko, my colleague, friend, teacher and just a close person

Roots and childhood

Konstantin Pavlovich was born near Kiev (Ukraine, when part of the USSR) in the village of Ivannitsa, Chernigov region. The ending '-ko' of his surname indicates Cossack origin. Konstantin Pavlovich loved Ukraine very much and considered it the centre of the universe, a place with an amazing climate and energy.

His parents were Ukrainians: a mechanic and a teacher. Already as a child, Buteyko was distinguished by his special character; he always did what he considered necessary. And his wise parents did not argue with him, constantly convinced of the independence and rationality of their son. "As a boy, I walked around naked, causing a lot of grief to my mother, but

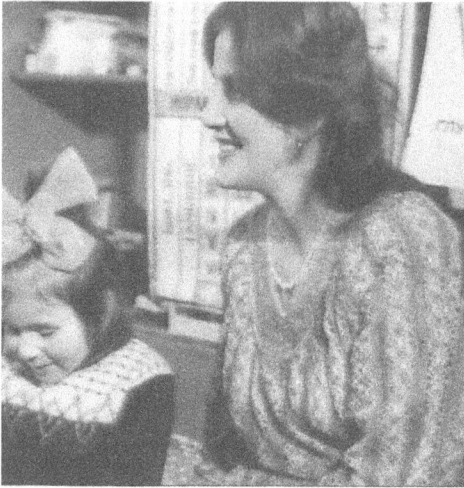

Dr Lyudmila Buteyko (Novozhilova), a frame from the film "Dr Buteyko's friends and enemies", Sverdlovsk Film Studio, 1988

I never got sick, and she stopped worrying about it," Buteyko used to say. A proud and independent child, he disliked overprotection and supervision. "What a strange boy I gave birth to!" his mother often said about him.

From childhood, Konstantin loved nature: "Everything was important to me; I studied every bug, every blade of grass, disappearing for hours in a field or forest." His grandmother had a great influence on the development of his personality. In her youth, she worked on the prince's estate, fell in love with Prince Svirsky and bore him two children. Her daughter became the mother of Konstantin Pavlovich. The grandmother knew all the medicinal herbs, knew how to heal, and let her inquisitive grandson into her secrets. After the death of the prince, his grandmother married a Cossack for the second time and at the age of 53 gave birth to another daughter. "I inherited my grandmother's analysis, logic and thinking," joked Buteyko. Then the family moved to Kiev.

His father cultivated in the future doctor a love of technology, and before the Second World War young Buteyko entered the Kiev Polytechnic Institute. He became highly proficient in technology and could diagnose the problems of a car by ear.

World War II

When the war began, Konstantin was a second-year student. During the intensive bombing of Kiev, he pulled the wounded from the ruins and rubble. Soon, he volunteered for the front line and went through the whole war without a single scratch! Twice he crossed the front line under bombard-ment. An accidental trip to the medical battalion determined his fate. There he saw blood, death and human suffering and realized the futility of killing.

He did not like to remember the war: "I saw the degradation of the human personality, the madness of war, the destruction of the best people. The bravest, the strongest were the first to attack, and the first to die. Then I realized that I needed to study the human body. We must learn to help! I decided to go to medical school in order to understand how everything works in a person." He returned to Moscow as a lieutenant, on assignment accompanied a train of trophy vehicles. For a whole year he was engaged in their service after the victory, at the same time preparing for the institute. It was then that his favourite expression appeared: «the most perfect ma-chine is the human organism!»

Sechenov First Moscow State Medical University

Buteyko entered the First Medical Institute named after Sechenov with the highest grades in all subjects. "I immediately set myself a global task – to defeat disease, to help humanity! I've seen too much grief." He was pur-suing his goal, receiving excellent marks, always doing brilliantly in any subject of the institute's programme.

In the second year, Konstantin Pavlovich asked the academician E. M. Tareev for permission to practise in the wards for incurable patients, where for the first time he saw how the nature of breathing changes in the last hours of a person's life. "Then, I could always accurately determine the time of the patient's passing from life by his breathing. And I have never been wrong! The nannies and nurses were afraid of me, they considered me a sorcerer ...", Dr Buteyko used to tell me. This realization haunted the young doctor's mind, and the search for truth began. Buteyko looked up all the available literature on the breathing in the libraries: "Many books were not even cut open, they were never opened, despite their answers to many global questions of medicine!", he told us. Indeed, before many scientists and physicians tried to understand the mechanism of the respiratory func-tion, they left a lot of works. Even Sechenov included studies of carbon dioxide for some time. Buteyko often referred to these authors, but did not forget to add that "many researchers followed the wrong path".

The discovery and first reactions

After graduating from the medical institute, the young scientist began work in Hospital № 24 at the Petrovsky Gates. There he began to form the idea of the presence of some connection between malignant hypertension and deep breathing, supported by the medical practice seen around him. As often happens, Buteyko fell ill with the very disease that he himself had been comprehensively studying for several years. Malignant hypertension overtook the young man. In search of health improvement, Buteyko practised yoga, various sports, tried to breathe deeply, considering, like everyone else around, that it was very useful. «I have travelled the standard path of common delusions with which patients come to me!»

Having an upper blood pressure of 300, Buteyko began to decrease his breathing, and the pressure dropped to 120. By performing an experiment on himself, Konstantin Pavlovich cured his hypertension! The simplicity of the method amazed him; he was shocked that no one had seen such an obvious pattern before. "I thought that if I could announce my discovery tomorrow, the whole world would know it and be saved!" But in reality it turned out differently: the teacher did not understand the student. Moreover, the audacity of the young doctor alerted the masters, aroused their

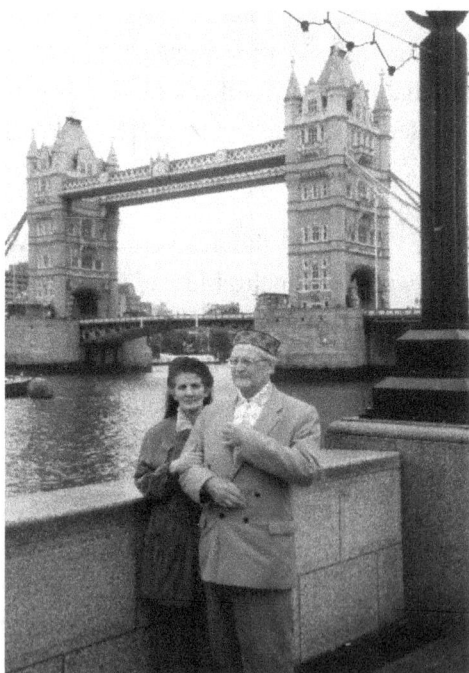

Dr Konstantin Buteyko and Dr Lyudmila Buteyko (Novozhilova), London, 2001

irritation and envy of the easy, as it seemed to them, success of the 'provincial upstart'.

Buteyko often recalled the fate of the Austrian obstetrician-gynecologist Ignaz Philipp Semmelweis, who discovered the nature of sepsis. He compared it with his own experience. Back in the 19th century, in Austria, the centre of world science and medicine, there was a university clinic where prostitutes gave birth and the students 'practised' on them. Eight out of ten of the women died from childbirth fever (postpartum sepsis). Semmelweis noticed that many students first went to the anatomical theatre to study, and then immediately went to the childbirth ward. Without washing their hands! At that time no one saw anything bad in this, there was no microscope yet, no one knew about the existence of microbes. But Semmelweis, 50 years before Louis Pasteur's discovery, suspected an obvious route of transmission. He made the students wash their hands thoroughly with chlorine as they left the anatomical theatre. As a result, the mortality rate of women in childbirth dropped significantly.

The Buteyko team and scientific discoveries

After a delayed reaction to the discovery in Moscow, the head of the Siberian branch of the USSR Academy of Sciences, mathematician M. A. Lavrentyev, invited Buteyko to Novosibirsk, to Akademgorodok. At that time, the best scientists of the country were invited to Akademgorodok. Budget funds were granted to set up a laboratory and to purchase expensive imported equipment. The young scientist was told to prove his discovery scientifically. Lavrentyev helped Buteyko considerably by buying diagnostic equipment in Denmark, and Buteyko used it extensively. The famous ballast-cardiograph or 'physiological harvester', as it was called in the laboratory, could forecast the programme of the heart for 15 years ahead! And a copyright certificate was obtained too.

Konstantin Pavlovich was obsessed with work and did not notice anything else. He gathered a circle of like-minded people around him and stayed till night-time in the laboratory, studying the problems of breathing. No one except Lavrentyev knew about the study. Moreover, the Institute of Mathematics, which he headed, provided comprehensive scientific support to the Buteyko Circle, backing up their research with mathematical calculations. Thus, each disease was illustrated with a chemical formula with mathematical dependence. The union of doctors and mathematicians turned out to be fruitful, bringing professional joy to like-minded scientists. For Buteyko and his team it was a happy time, full of scientific flight, search and joy of discovery.

Persecution

In August 1968, an order came to close the laboratory, to dissolve the scientific staff. Immediately, a group of unknown people broke into the building of the institute at night and destroyed the laboratory: they tore up medical records, scattered papers, chopped up a unique physiological combine with an axe, which alone cost half a million dollars. At that time Buteyko was in Moscow when he received an urgent telegram: "Trouble! Come back immediately!" He flew to Novosibirsk and rushed to his laboratory. As his colleagues recall, "He entered and immediately became grey-haired!" This man with colossal willpower did not show his shock any more. The laboratory staff managed to save from barbaric destruction only the medical history of the patients who had passed through the physiological combine.

This was the reaction of the authorities to the brilliant discovery of Dr Buteyko. Because how can you treat people without drugs? What will hospitals, institutes, pharmacological factories do? Directly closing the laboratory would be too provocative, so it was accused of 'scientific unreasonableness'. Konstantin Pavlovich understood everything. Everything seemed over – he was left without work, without employees, without support. He went to Moscow, tried to discover the truth, but without success. Three times they tried to hide him in a psychiatric hospital, but each time there were not enough signatures for the resolution. Two doctors signed, but a third one did not! His conscience did not allow.

People's hope for the Buteyko Method and our first meeting

But the doctor was not alone for long. The fame of the author of a unique treatment method, of hundreds of cured patients was beyond the control of officials. People were trying to reach Buteyko. As before, he went to the library, "corrected" dissertations for friends, only now he had to work with patients from home. Sick people were coming from all over the world, hoping to find help and recover.

This is how I met him. I was seriously ill with a hormone-dependent form of bronchial asthma, and even a tumor in the chest – cystic mastopathy. At the age of 29, I was a disabled person of the first group. Huge doses of hormones, a moustache, a beard, a weight of 120 kilograms … I was constantly suffocating; all the ambulances in Moscow knew me, because I spent most of the year in hospitals. My situation was depressing; all my relatives and friends tried to help me somehow, looking for any means of salvation. Then in 1968 I came across a newspaper article about Buteyko. I realized that this was my chance, and immediately wrote him a letter, addressed to 'Novosibirsk. To Doctor Buteyko.' But with no known address, my letter was returned. Hope melted with it. But once I obtained the exact address of Buteyko, with great difficulty, I wrote again. Time passed and suddenly I received a telegram: 'I will be passing through Moscow. I can visit you.' On 9 February 1969, the doorbell rang. Every year I celebrate this date that turned my life upside down, my second birthday.

The first thing I noticed was the unusually intense gaze of a tall, stately man. He said that his first impression of me was depressing: "I saw a dying woman in front of me." This strange doctor took out a stopwatch and said, "Now we are measuring how much you cannot breathe!" I was upset because the proposal seemed to me, to put it mildly, strange. My pause at that moment was very small. Convinced of this, he said that I was breathing deeply, and it was making me sick. He patiently explained the danger of my situation, described the way to salvation. His words about breathing barely reached me; I almost regretted this useless meeting. Am I breathing deeply? I cannot breathe at all! I'm choking! But Buteyko kept saying the same thing: "You need to breathe less!" he said brusquely.

Noticing my bewilderment, he drew a breathing pattern, and recommended small pauses between exhalation and inhalation. I still keep this drawing. And then, I kept listening in a daze. Buteyko read my thoughts: "Okay, is there anyone else at home?" "My son," I answered. "Call him!"

The 9-year-old Andrey came in. Buteyko began to explain something quietly to him, and then, turning sharply in my direction, said: "Your mother is very sick. If you want to save her, try to explain to her everything that I have just told you, so that she will really understand." And he left.

Further collaboration and observation

After our second meeting, we began to live and work together. Buteyko believed in me. I myself had not yet fully recovered, but I inspired others with my confidence in success. He saw my attitude to the method and marked common interests and positions. Then for 34 years we lived side by side, and every day I saw something new and exciting in him, until he died on 2 May 2003. Even five days before, on 27 April, people from the East came to him, and for four hours they talked with inspiration about philosophy and the method, of course. Visitors were always amazed at his knowledge.

Immediately after we met, Buteyko invited me to a lecture for doctors, which shocked me. His knowledge was extraordinary! In general, I have not missed any of his lectures. In all the years of our life together, it was impossible to tear myself away from his speeches. And today, reading his works, all the time I notice something new. When Buteyko first told me about the method, the world turned upside down for me! Such simple, obvious things seemed to me a salvation for many suffering people. Buteyko himself was a very unusual person; it is impossible to compare him with anyone. His intellect, attitude to people, value system – everything was unique in him. He had his own opinion on everything, his own reasoned answer to any question.

Konstantin Pavlovich used to repeat that a doctor, a scientist, must trust his intuition. But he not only studied brilliantly and received the highest marks from the best professors in the country; he was also tirelessly engaged in scientific work. Of course, a sudden flash of genius is necessary

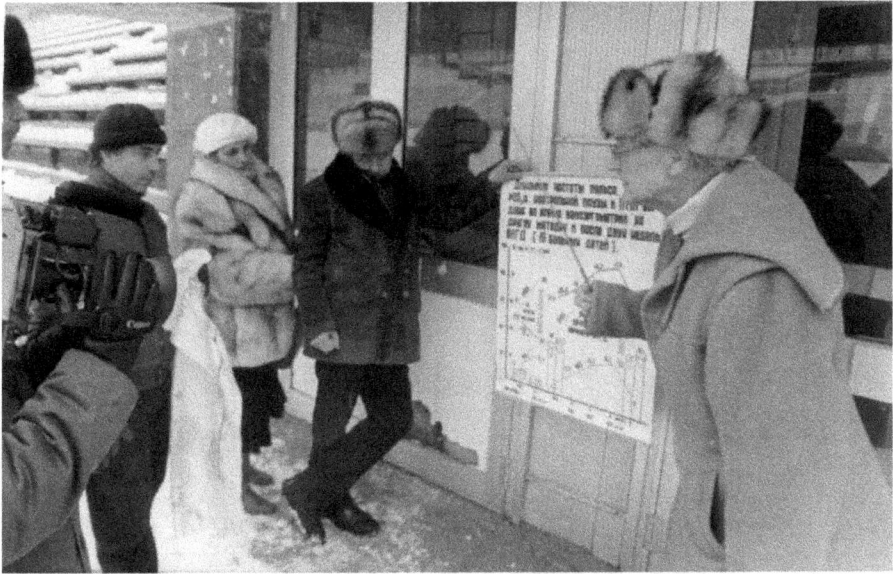

Dr Buteyko before the start of one of his public lectures, mid-1980s, Novosibirsk. He is demonstrating one of the famous tables of the dependence of bicycle ergometry indicators and the dynamics of pCO2.

for any scientific discovery, but behind this flash there is always gigantic hard labour. "Nothing comes from nothing!" It is a pity that today, besides us and his followers, Buteyko's scientific background, his archive, is of little interest to anyone. This is surprising. Official medicine continues to depart from the Buteyko Method, as if he were some kind of charlatan … I repeat once again, Buteyko is not a healer, not a medium; he is a brilliant doctor and an outstanding scientist who saved hundreds of thousands of people, and that's it!

Buteyko did not like teaching. He simply gave out his recommendations, and if the person immediately understood, the work continued. By contrast, I love teaching and he always told me, "You are the only one who can teach the method correctly!" Buteyko loved those patients who were 'catching on the fly', quick learners who were interested in a quick result. When a 'difficult' patient came and for a long time could not understand what was said, he always called me: "Here, your patient has come!"

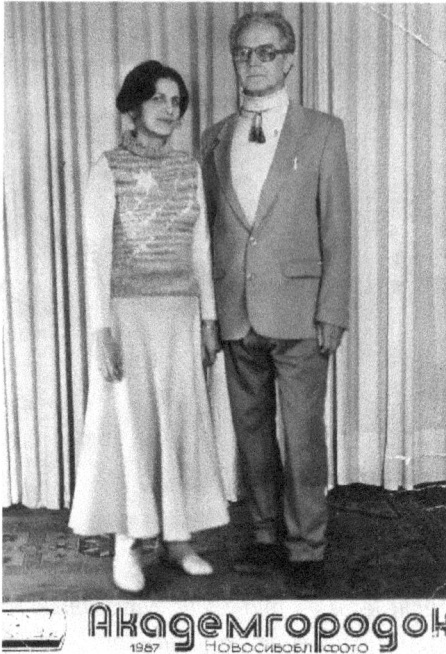

Dr Konstantin Buteyko with Dr Lyudmila Buteyko (Novozhilova), Novosibirsk, 1987

I was surprised at my patience. But I had been in a similar position: I remember that previously I did not immediately understand the technique! For almost a whole year I had only a short pause, and once I caught a cold, started coughing, and at night I had a severe attack. I called an ambulance, stood by the window, waited and thought: "And my patients know nothing about my asthma attacks! I, apparently, do not fully understand everything." Then suddenly I felt the movement of my respiratory muscles; I relaxed them and the attack disappeared. Buteyko observed it all, got up from his chair and said, "Well, finally, you have understood. There will be no more asthma then!" I experienced the effect of the method in myself, and now I knew exactly how to explain the problem to people. So patients come to me for this.

Organ weakness and deep breathing are inherited. I always draw the attention of my patients to this, unmistakably enumerating for them all the 'baggage' of hereditary elements and diseases. Buteyko taught me this. In general, he always gave great importance to diagnostics: a thorough examination, and only then prescriptions and an individual approach to every patient – this was Buteyko's credo. I was always amazed at his attitude towards any patient, towards the diagnosis. He did this clearly, explaining in detail the cause of the disease and its possible development. He gave the patient a picture of the past, present and future. Everyone sat with their mouths open in fascination! Everyone always listened to him, and it was impossible otherwise: he was so convincing, sincere! It was evident that he knew what he was talking about, knew it deeply. It inspired people immensely.

Buteyko saved me from the tumour. It happened due to his knowledge, experience, understanding of physiological processes. I was registered at the oncological dispensary, and when I was once again invited for examination, the doctor almost fell off his chair – there was no tumour! "What did I prescribe you?!" he stuttered. He had prescribed the strongest hormones. And then I told him about Buteyko. He was an unusual doctor, this oncologist. He thought for a moment and then said, "So the tumour went away because of this." Then I went to the radiologist, who had previously seen my pictures with practically no lungs left. Seeing such dramatic changes, this doctor was not at all surprised, as if she saw this result every day and she did not bother to ask me where to send her suffering patients. This shocks me. Unfortunately, doctors today very rarely send patients to us. This is strange.

Opening the Buteyko Clinic in Moscow

Meanwhile, the interest in Buteyko was enormous. Konstantin P. Buteyko lived in Moscow, and the patients were coming to his home. The authorities forgot about him; the medical world pretended that there was no such doctor as Buteyko. Then there was Novosibirsk. I constantly flew to him and watched his moral sufferings. No wonder he compared his medical fate with Semmelweis; many things were too similar. The apartment in Novosibirsk was always filled with visitors, patients and journalists. The city hotel was overflowing with people who wanted to meet the magical doctor; the name of Buteyko became a legend. People told each other about their own healing and went to find Konstantin Pavlovich themselves. Even in Crimea, where we went every year, we were constantly tracked down by sick people looking for healing by the Buteyko Method. And Buteyko never refused anyone. Wherever he was invited to give a speech, he accepted: at enterprises, in clinics, in kindergartens. And he continued to teach and prepare Buteyko Methodists, preferring to 'make' them out of his patients who he himself had healed. Thus passed the 1970s.

At the beginning of Perestroika, the wall of silence collapsed: journalists longed for interviews with Dr Buteyko, film crews went to his flat from all over the country. Many articles came out. In 1981, another approbation of the method took place, and in 1983 he received the second copyright certificate for it. In 1988, the dream of Konstantin Pavlovich was finally realized: with the active support of the regional authorities, the Buteyko Clinic was opened in Moscow on 3rd Vladimirskaya Street. How happy he was! That's how it all turned out: they brought me a 3-month-old baby girl with bedsores and shortness of breath. She turned out to be a relative of the director of the Prozhektor plant, who suggested that we organize a medical cooperative at his base. So the first seal of approval for the Clinic was a factory seal. Later, a permit to organize the Breathing cooperative was also signed. The flow of people was enormous. Konstantin Pavlovich was resurrected, his face became happy – people needed him!

Deep breathing is the cause of all human troubles

Buteyko considered deep breathing to be the cause of all human troubles: not only diseases, but also wars, social conflict, lies and violence. Deep breathing is unnatural, uncomfortable for a person, hence increased aggressiveness, anger, envy and hatred. Dr Buteyko himself listened to any person, never refused to help patients. A real doctor. And he demanded the same attitude towards people from his students (the methodists). He used to tell me, "Never lie. If you feel awkward, better keep silent, leave, but don't lie." People like Buteyko are the people of the future; maybe they will save the world someday. He was always against wars, enmity and disagreements.

Before starting a family, he recommended his patients to check on the health of the older generation of the future wife or husband. Buteyko had his own system of working with pregnant women. He believed that for a successful conception, a woman must achieve a pause in breathing for 180 seconds! Only then can she give birth to an absolutely healthy child. The newborn overcomes any gene dependence or bad inheritance. I saw such families in Novosibirsk, with children born by this method. These are the people of the future!

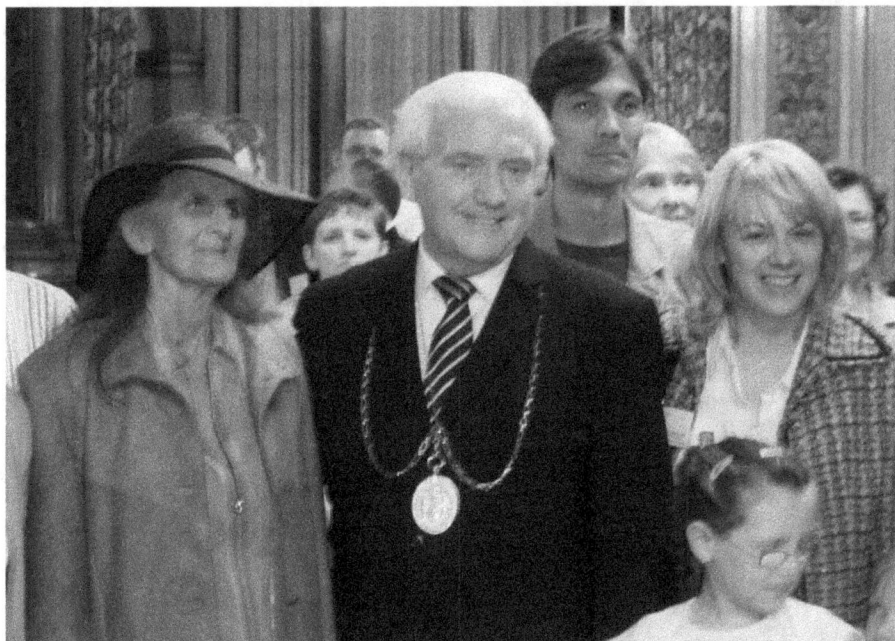
Dr Lyudmila Buteyko (Novozhilova) and Dr Jill McGown at Glasgow City Hall, 2005

"I did everything I could!"

He was tough in character, terribly principled, stubborn and absolutely obsessed with his goal. Konstantin P. Buteyko respected personality, loved justice, considered retribution for bad deeds inevitable. He passionately believed that the future belongs to positive people, that the fate of humanity depends on them, and the preponderance of negative forces leads to war. He used to repeat that nature forgives people nothing. "If you have done a bad deed, you will get what you deserve", he was always saying. He spoke everything directly face to face, never hid the diagnosis from the patient, considered it necessary to provide complete information. Sometimes he said things that were unpleasant for the public, things that people prefer not to notice in themselves.

Konstantin P. Buteyko did not know what fear and betrayal was, and if he walked towards something, he did not turn away.

This inflexibility played a critical role in his career as a scientist. In Soviet times, as you know, they did not like 'upstarts', pioneers and geniuses, especially those who spoke the truth.

His life cannot be called easy and happy. But he was happy with his victories, his cured patients. His life, and especially his career, were rather tragic, probably like that of any large-scale scientist. In recent years, he often repeated: "Why are you looking at me, are you discussing my life? You had better read my works, take a look at my discoveries …
I did everything I could!"

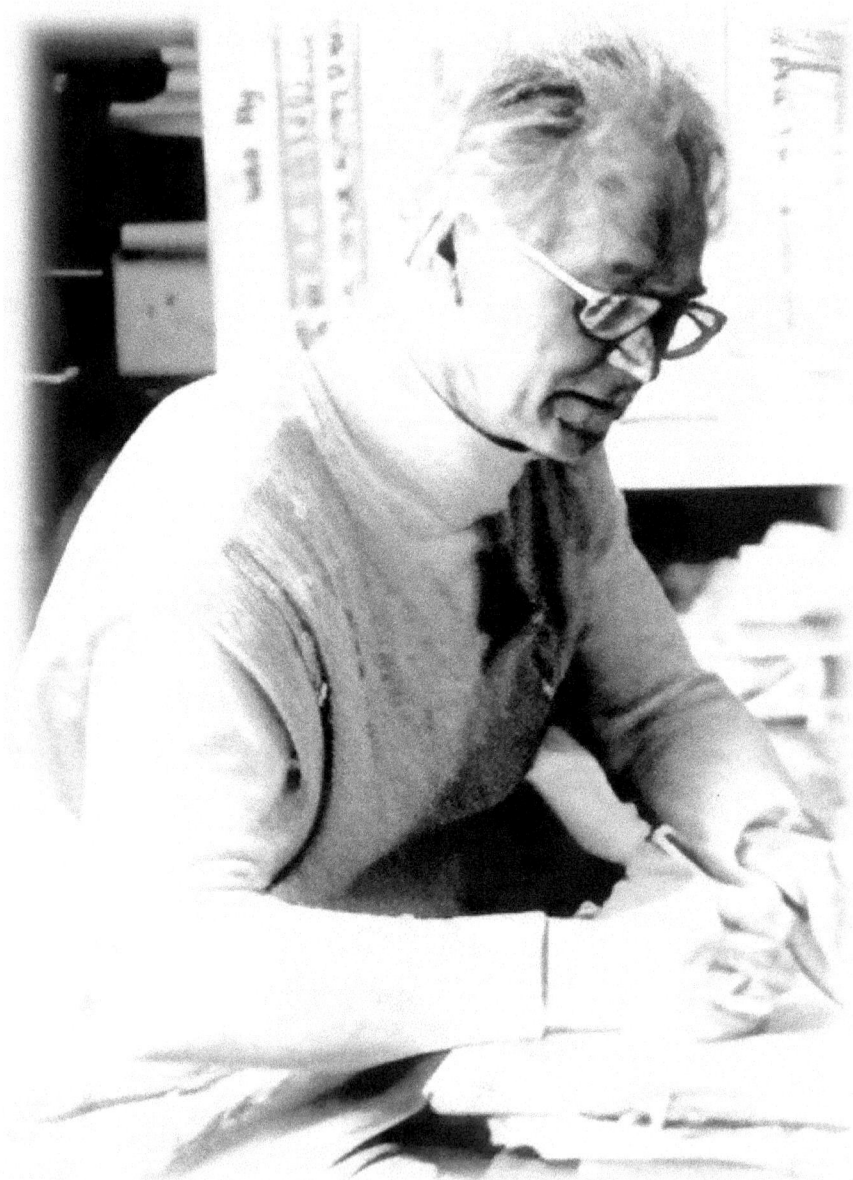

Dr Konstantin P. Buteyko, 1970s

Dr Konstantin P. Buteyko: some aphorisms from lectures, collected by Dr Andrey E. Novozhilov

Anna Novozhilova

Director of the programme 'Genuine Buteyko breathing techniques from Primary Sources for Foreigners'

Certified Buteyko Method specialist of the Buteyko Clinic in Moscow (est. 1987)

"It is necessary to eliminate the causes of deep breathing, and not just train the breathing itself.

Deep breathing as a cause of disease has its own causes. It is necessary to look for the reasons for deep breathing, then you will not have to do breathing exercises for the rest of your life.

Deep breathing will cause illness until you find and eliminate the causes of the deepest breathing.

Therefore, in order to defeat the disease, it is necessary to clean the brain, not the rectum."

"If someone had told me that I would need to teach people how to decrease breathing, I would not believe it."

"It takes 30 seconds to test the validity of the scientific discovery we made 30 years ago: suggest to an asthmatic to hyperventilate and you will see him choking with an asthma attack; suggest that he reduces breathing and you will see the attack relieved. The cause of an asthma attack is hyperventilation of the lungs. No one mentioned it before our scientific research. And so I have been asking scientists for 30 years to spend 30 seconds to check this (1986)."

"The main reason for deep breathing is the deception of medicine: breathe deeper – more oxygen! So the entire uneducated public is about to die in the pursuit of oxygen, of which there is already quite enough in the arterial blood. And the funny thing in this situation is that there is no way to add more oxygen there!"

"Breathing is atomic energy; playing with breathing leads to death!"

"Who was the fool who first said, 'Breathe deeper - more oxygen'? For almost 40 years I can't find whether anyone has checked this statement with an elementary measurement. This has not been tested on a single person, after all! And everyone, like parrots, repeat, 'Breathe deeper – it's useful!'"

"The reason why modern civilization will perish was discovered by me on 7 October 1952."

"Computers have no intelligence, they cannot open anything. They do only what the human mind has determined for them. The computer does not have the freedom of thought necessary for creativity and scientific discovery."

"My method is extremely simple: reduce your breathing, you don't have to do anything else. Bronchial obstruction and coughing, choking or high blood pressure are eliminated by themselves when breathing is normalized, because all these diseases are compensatory reactions aimed at normalizing breathing and respiratory homeostasis."

"Why does my method seem hard? Because causal thinking is lost."

"I was 100-200 years late. In past centuries, they were still looking for the cause of any disease: the cause of plague, cholera and malaria. Once found and understood, the disease was eliminated. And the cause of heart attack, stroke, cancer, allergies had not been found. I found it, but too late: causal thinking has degenerated. I speak out loudly about it but nobody hears."

"Any ignorant and incompetent manipulations with breathing only make it deeper and kill us."

"Nowadays medicine teaches the population to breathe deeply; it teaches people deep breathing."

"The more medicine, the more pills, more beds, more death."

"A deep-breathing mother gives birth to a deep-breathing baby. In accordance with the laws of physiology, such a child is doomed to get sick, because the organism dies from deep breathing within 10 minutes or compensatory mechanisms arise, on the basis of which diseases arise."

"I discovered the Law of Death: the deeper the breathing, the more severe is the illness and the closer the death of the organism."

"Everyone trains in deep breathing – this is a terrible nonsense. There is no more stupid prejudice than this prejudice. I have said a million times and I repeat it again: arterial blood is always completely saturated with oxygen, so deep breathing cannot add even more oxygen."

"No devices, simulators and other nonsense are able to reduce breathing; they cannot normalize the respiratory function; these devices are a deception for people. You need to feel your breathing. It is necessary to reduce breathing by one quarter. Do not reduce breathing too much. I am 100-200 years late. In past centuries, they were still looking for the cause of the disease."

Some aphorisms about the Buteyko Method, by Dr Andrey E. Novozhilov

Anna Novozhilova

Director of the programme 'Genuine Buteyko breathing techniques from Primary Sources for Foreigners'

Certified Buteyko Method specialist of the Buteyko Clinic in Moscow (est. 1987)

The Buteyko Method in the words of experienced specialists

"An 'old' or classic Buteyko practitioner will never say that the Buteyko Method is a set of breathing exercises; but that the Buteyko Method is a healthy lifestyle and a huge complex of knowledge."

The Buteyko Method is not a set of breathing exercises

"It is impossible to reduce the Buteyko Method as a treatment system exclusively to performing breathing exercises.

Dr Buteyko always forbade calling the Buteyko Method a set of breathing exercises.

Every 'old' or classic Buteyko practitioner who studied with Dr Buteyko himself, and then worked for many years, will always say that 'The essence of the Buteyko Method as a method of treatment is to normalize breathing, respiratory homeostasis; this is the key condition for health.'

It is possible to normalize the respiratory function with the help of sports, or with the help of correct posture, or with the help of fine sensitivity to breathing, and you never know what other ways exist.

Therefore, the Buteyko Method is both sports and correct posture, which most people have long forgotten about, and the formation of a fine sensitivity to breathing and much more, not only breathing exercises.

Our organism is a so-called open system, the viability of which is ensured by maintaining the constancy of the internal environment or homeostasis. So breathing exercises will be useful if they normalize respiratory homeostasis.

Today, many people talk about the benefits of breathing exercises, but no one talks about homeostasis, so almost no one understands the physiological meaning and benefits of breathing exercises from a scientific point of view.

If the teacher does not talk about the importance of breathing exercises for the normalization of respiratory homeostasis, it means that this teacher does not know physiology well and does not understand the role of breathing in maintaining health."

Why do children get sick?

"The cause of a child's illness is the deep breathing of the parents."

"The child's health will always depend on the parent's Control Pause while the child lives with them."

"Raising children begins from the first day of pregnancy, and the health of the child begins from the high Control Pause of their future parents."

Why do people get sick?

"The cause of an adult's illness is their own deep breathing and nothing more and no one more.

Remove deep breathing, and there will be no diseases.

If you cannot remove deep breathing, then look for the reasons for your deep breathing and remove them – and there will be no diseases.

The best way to remove deep breathing is relaxation till there is a slight hunger for air - which means without changing the pattern of breathing."

To reduce breathing is a highly creative sort of art

"To reduce breathing is a kind of art. Many people are born with the talent to feel their breath and reduce the depth of breathing. This talent, like any other and like any art, must be developed and directed in the right way."

Delicate sensitivity to breathing is not mindless breathing exercises

"The Buteyko breathing technique forms an understanding of how breathing changes in different life situations. But the Buteyko breathing technique in most cases does not sufficiently normalize the work of the breathing system, because it is performed for only a limited time. For successful treatment, preservation and improvement of health, we must ourselves, without the constant implementation of the Buteyko breathing technique itself, normalize the work of the respiratory system using our delicate sensitivity to breathing and our understanding of how breathing changes, and using various methods of fine-tuning of breathing."

Disease formula and health formula

"Buteyko not only spoke the Law of Death: the deeper the breathing, the closer the death of the organism; he also spoke the Law of Life: breathlessness is immortality. Disease Formula and Health Formula."

"Dr K. Buteyko discovered Deep Breathing Disease and proposed to unify/ merge 150 diseases into one group based on the common cause of their occurrence. An interesting fact is that these 150 diseases account for almost 90% of illness cases of people in the modern world; therefore, their successful treatment with the Buteyko breathing technique (BBT) creates a kind of panacea effect, although there is deep scientific research and a number of fundamental scientific discoveries behind the Buteyko breathing technique (BBT)."

"Dr K. Buteyko created the Formula of Health: reducing the breathing means healing and health, and, having decoded the secrets of yogic health and longevity from a scientific point of view, Dr K. Buteyko announced the Law of Life: breathlessness is immortality. The words of Indian yogis, several thousand years old, have received scientific explanation and confirmation. Breathlessness here is rather invisibility, spirituality, ephemerality of breathing. It was expressed by the Chinese philosopher Lao Tzu accurately 2,500 years ago: the breathing of a perfect person is as if he does not breathe."

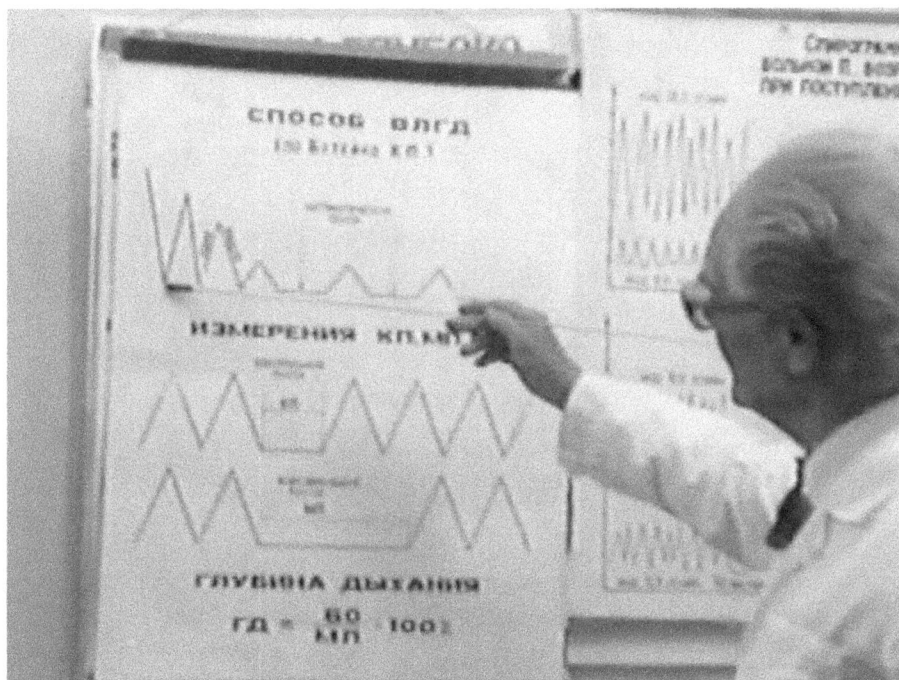

Dr Buteyko explains the formula of perfection proposed by the Chinese philosopher Lao Tzu 2,500 years ago: "A perfect man breathes as if he is not breathing."

Dr Buteyko explains the change in the pattern of breathing during a decrease in the depth of breathing.

The best way to remove deep breathing is relaxation until a slight hunger for air. Slight hunger for air, it means without changing the pattern of breathing.

A change in the pattern of breathing during the reduction of breathing by relaxation.

A frame from the video recording of Dr Buteyko's lecture, in the 1990s.

The essence of the Buteyko Method by Claudia Schyia

Claudia Schyia

Certified Buteyko Method specialist

Cologne, Germany

Normal breathing: the key to good health and athletic performance

Dear friends of the genuine Buteyko Method, for 40 years I have been looking for a way to cure bronchial asthma and no longer be dependent on medication.

I researched numerous possible treatments including yoga, proper nutrition, sports, a healthy lifestyle and much more, but the asthma did not subside and did not give up.

Medical doctors told me directly and honestly that they did not know how to cure asthma, that asthma could not be cured with medication, that this disease was with me for life.

One day I heard about Dr Buteyko from Russia, who had invented a non-drug way to treat asthma through breathing techniques, known as the Buteyko Method.

I learned the Buteyko Method, the Buteyko breathing techniques, and my asthma improved significantly.

I have stopped taking medication and now I've been living for several years without asthma and almost without medication.

Buteyko breathing techniques are only one part of the Buteyko Method

By the way, looking ahead a bit, it should be said that the Buteyko Method is not a set of breathing exercises.

Here it is necessary to clarify that Buteyko breathing techniques are only one part of the Buteyko Method as a drug-free method of treatment.

Another part of the Buteyko Method is a large complex of critically important knowledge, which in some cases can provide excellent healing results even without the use of breathing techniques.

For example, did you know that asthma or high blood pressure can be completely cured with the help of sport, but on the condition of normal breathing during sport?

I studied the Buteyko Method, Buteyko breathing techniques under the guidance of Dr Andrey Novozhilov.

Dr Andrey Novozhilov is the co-inventor of the Buteyko Method and chief physician of the Buteyko Clinic in Moscow.

The medical clinic in Moscow was personally organized by Dr Buteyko in 1987 and has been successfully treating patients with asthma for more than 30 years.

Why is it interesting to be a certified Buteyko Method specialist?

The Buteyko Method interested me and inspired me so much that I decided to get trained as a certified specialist and start teaching the Buteyko Method to other people.

I noticed that when I explain the Buteyko Method and Buteyko breathing techniques to other people, my asthma recedes from me step-by-step and goes away.

Dr Novozhilov explained to me that teaching other people helps you understand the Buteyko Method, helps you gain new experience in the treatment of asthma, so teaching other people always greatly helps you to recover. I felt that teaching other people the Buteyko Method was a condition of my own recovery from asthma in terms of logic, in terms of physiology and even, if you like, some mysticism.

A simple and easy explanation of the essence of the Buteyko Method

The ability to explain the essence of the Buteyko Method is based solely on personal experience of its application

I asked Dr Novozhilov, who treated my asthma, how best to explain to people the essence of the Buteyko Method as a treatment method?

How easy is it to explain that the Buteyko Method can cure asthma completely, but not medicines?

Dr Novozhilov told me that the main thing in the presentation is your own experience with Buteyko. It will sound sincere and true.

He repeated the words of Dr Buteyko: If you are not a doctor, then tell the patient only your own experience of training and recovery and tell very little about medical theory, because the patient will immediately sense that you are not a doctor.

It is necessary to talk very little about the scientific and medical part of the Buteyko Method, but to talk a lot and share your Buteyko studies, talk about successes and defeats along the way.

To understand the essence of the Buteyko Method, it is necessary to remember the definition of what HEALTH is

After that, Dr Novozhilov said, in order to understand why the Buteyko Method is able to completely cure asthma, it is necessary to remember what HEALTH is from the point of view of medicine and the science of physiology.

Dr Novozhilov told me a short story about what HEALTH is from the point of view of the science of physiology, how to maintain or restore health if you have any disease.

Physiology is a science that studies the laws of the life of our organism.

Our organism is a large complex of so-called functional systems: for example, the respiratory system, muscular system, nervous system, cardiovascular system, digestive system and others. The work of each of them maintains constant physiological values, the so-called constants.

For example, the organism's temperature is a constant: always the same, no matter where we are, in Africa or at the North Pole.

Blood pressure is a physiological constant and is constant, as is blood sugar and so on; there are many other physiological constants that ensure the normal functioning of our organism.

If the constant changes, then the organism dies.

But special compensatory mechanisms arise and begin to work before death in order to normalize the disturbed constants.

Usually, these compensatory mechanisms look like habitual diseases: bronchospasm and suffocation, vasospasm and increased blood pressure, and others.

For example, in the middle of the last century, scientists conducted some famous experiments whose results were explained only by Dr Buteyko.

A healthy dog was forced to breathe deeply and the dog died after 10 minutes. Scientists could not explain the reason for the death of the dog.

Only Dr Buteyko, 30 years later, explained that the dog died as the result of a change in gas constants, as a result of spasm of the vessels of the heart muscle. This was the cause of the massive heart attack and death of the dog.

The same story is often found in professional sports.

We hear in news programmes that runners have died on the track or ice hockey players during their game. Recently, information appeared in the news that a quite famous actor bought an exercise bicycle to get back in shape after being sick, and he ended up dead on this bicycle. There was a huge public response and panic because people thought the problem was in the exercise bicycle, while the real problem was the actor's breathing.

The reason for their death is very simple.

Prolonged hyperventilation in an athlete leads to a change in gas constants and the emergence of compensatory mechanisms, the work of which tends to normalize the changed constants. The organism can die as a result of a violation of gas constants or as a result of the work of compensatory mechanisms: as a result of vasospasm or bronchospasm.

For example, the organism raises its temperature upon contact with a virus in order to destroy the virus. But the organism itself can die from this high temperature.

Let us return to the question of what is health.

What is health?

Health is the state of the organism when all key constants correspond to the physiological norm: the organism's temperature is normal, its blood pressure is normal, blood sugar is normal, oxygen and CO_2 are normal, and so on.

The first characteristic of health is the normal constants that ensure the normal functioning of the organism.

The second characteristic of health is that all the functional systems of the organism which ensure the maintenance of constants within the normal range are working normally.

What is disease?

A disease is a condition that has arisen as a result of a change in specific constants and the work of compensatory mechanisms that seek to return the constants to normal.

What is diagnostics?

Diagnostics means the search for constants specific to a given disease, the change in which caused this disease. For example, a change in the insulin constant that leads to diabetes.

What is treatment?

Treatment is the process of returning the constants to normal, the normalization of the constants specific to the given disease. Normalization of constants allows you to eliminate the action of compensatory mechanisms, the work of which also tends to normalize the changing constants.

For example, normalization of the CO_2 constant in the lungs eliminates bronchospasm, which is a compensatory mechanism that also tends to normalize CO_2 in the lungs.

If the CO_2 constant in the lungs changes, then bronchial obstruction and bronchospasm occur.

If the O_2 constant changes at the level of metabolism (metabolic hypoxia), then there is a vasospasm and an increase in blood pressure.

Bronchospasm and an asthma attack, vasospasm and increased blood pressure are specific compensatory mechanisms that arise as a result of changes in gas constants in the lungs, in the blood, in cells and whose work tends to normalize respiratory homeostasis.

Respiratory homeostasis is the constancy of the gas composition of blood and cells.

Reversible bronchial obstruction, bronchospasm or high blood pressure cannot be cured with drugs, because bronchospasm and vasospasm are not diseases in the usual sense of the word; but they are compensatory mechanisms that will work until the gas constants in the lungs (CO_2 constant) or in organism cells (O_2 constant) are normalized or the organism will die.

Dr Buteyko opened some keys to health and pointed out that it is possible to cure asthma or blood pressure without drugs, but on condition that the gas constants are normalized.

Why the Buteyko Method is not a set of breathing exercises

Here it should be said that there are natural mechanisms for the normalization of gas constants.

Dr Buteyko's scientific research explained how these mechanisms work and allowed us to incorporate them into the Buteyko Method to use as a treatment. Therefore, the Buteyko Method cannot be reduced to breathing techniques only.

For example, physical activity is a natural mechanism for normalizing gas constants and respiratory homeostasis. Here it is important to understand that muscle activity, exercise or sports normalize the work of the respiratory system and gas constants only when breathing through the nose.

The famous Buteyko breathing techniques are only one part of the Buteyko Method as a method of treatment. These techniques are usually used only at the initial stage of the treatment of severe patients.

Another part of the Buteyko Method is a large complex of knowledge about our breathing, about the laws of physiology, the knowledge of which helps prevent the occurrence of many diseases that cannot be cured with medicines: asthma, allergies, chronic rhinitis, high blood pressure, diabetes and many others.

Normal breathing, according to Buteyko, during sport allows you to increase sports endurance and increase sports results.

The Buteyko Method and knowledge of the basic laws of respiratory physiology provide answers to the questions of how to exercise safely and effectively, how to cure asthma or allergies successfully with the help of dosed sports physical activity under the control of breathing.

The Buteyko Method answers the question of how to prevent an asthma attack during a night's sleep, or how to prevent a coughing fit as a result of a long emotional conversation.

For example, did you know that it is possible to cure chronic runny nose, allergies and bronchial asthma or high blood pressure with the help of sport, provided that breathing is normal during the sport?

Normal breathing is when the gas constants in the lungs, blood, cells of the organism correspond to the physiological norm.

Therefore, it is necessary to measure the key CO_2 constant before and after sport in order to know for sure that breathing was normal and the respiratory system worked normally during sport.

I will gladly tell you about it.

Lung ventilation criteria									
Health Status	Breathing pattern	Degree of violation	pCO₂ in alveoli.		Control pause	Maximum pause	Auto pause	Respiratory Rate (per minute)	Pulse (per minute)
			%	Mm Hg					
Super hardiness	Shallow breathing	V	7,5	54	90	180	16	3	48
		IV	7,4	53	75	150	12	4	50
		III	7,3	52	60	120	9	5	52
		II	7,1	51	50	100	7	6	55
		I	6,8	48	40	80	5	7	57
Norm			6,5	46	30	60	4	8	60
Disease	Hyperventilation of the lungs	I	6,0	43	25	50	3	10	65
		II	5,5	40	20	40	2	12	70
		III	5,0	36	15	30	1	15	75
		IV	4,5	32	10	20	-	20	80
		V	4,0	28	5	10	-	26	90

Dr Buteyko's famous chart for determining the degree
of deep breathing disease

Dr Buteyko's table to measure the CO_2 constant in the lungs

Dr Buteyko developed a unique table to measure the CO_2 constant in the lungs in order to identify breathing patterns and health status.

The table shows average parameters at rest.

Dr Buteyko developed this table after his laboratory in Siberia (Institute of Experimental Biology and Medicine, Siberian Branch of the USSR Academy of Sciences, Novosibirsk) was attacked to deliberately destroy his work.

With the help of this table, you can easily recognize a trend of your breathing habits (hyperventilation or normal, shallow breathing) and state of health. You only need to measure the Control Pause (CP) when you wake up in the morning and are still in bed. If you perform the CP measurement correctly, you will get a solid indication of your state of health, because you cannot control your breathing while you are asleep (source: *Breathing by Buteyko. Practice and Theory*, by Dr Andrey Novozhilov).

Dr Buteyko classified health status into 3 categories: The Norm (Good Health), Super Hardiness and Disease.

The norm: good health

The highlighted box in the table represents the norm: A healthy person has a morning CP of 30 seconds or a maximum pause of 60 seconds. The carbon dioxide level in the lungs corresponds to the physiological norm of 6.5%, which ensures that the gas constants in the blood and cells of the organism correspond to the physiological norm as well. People in this category have normal breathing and good health. The metabolism and immune system are normal.

If we look at how our breathing changes as the gas constants normalize, we will see the following interesting facts.

If we look at our breathing at rest, we will see that the Automatic Pause (after exhalation, before the next breath) of 1 second appears when the morning CP reaches 15 seconds. Many people experience this automatic cessation of breathing at rest.

The duration of the automatic pause after exhalation increases when the morning CP increases, so the respiratory rate can decrease significantly to 2 to 3 breaths per minute if the automatic pause reaches values of 15 to 20 seconds.

The heart rate (pulse) also decreases.

It should be said that the numbers in the table are approximate figures and show a trend or a possible course of events, but are not absolutely accurate. The numbers in this table are very individual and have a personal difference, but the trend is the same for all people. For example, in some asthmatic patients, choking attacks stop at 15 seconds CP, but some asthmatic patients sometimes have asthma attacks at 40 seconds CP; however, we see a trend of decreasing numbers of choking attacks with increasing CP.

Accurate figures are used in scientific research, but it is important for us to show a trend or pattern of recovery.

Several versions of this table can be found in the sources, where different numbers are indicated. These tables were published as a result of researches conducted by Dr Buteyko himself in different periods. Therefore, now, in order to avoid discrepancies or disagreements, it makes sense to talk rather about a trend, and not about exact numbers. And once again it should be pointed out that the numbers are very personal for each patient. For example, some patients no longer have asthma attacks at a CP of 15 seconds, and some people stop having asthma attacks when they have a CP of 30 to 40 seconds.

Super hardiness

Dr Buteyko divided this health level into 5 categories.

The table tells us that the depth and frequency of breathing decrease as CO_2 levels increase; but this is a trend, not exact numbers.

Thus, we reach the famous formula for the perfect person (Lao Tzu, 2,500 years ago): "The breath of a perfect man is as if he were not breathing."

Category I–III: People in this category have shallow breathing and are very healthy. The carbon dioxide level in the lungs has increased from 6.5% (modern physiological norm) to 6.8-7.3%.

Dr Buteyko added that at the higher end of the CP time measurements (40 seconds and more), individuals demonstrate a high level of athletic endurance, they need only a few hours of sleep, are free of viral infections and diseases, and have a lower pulse and breathing rate at rest. Their metabolism and immune system will automatically revert to normal.

Category IV–V: People on the far higher end of the scale with a CP of 75 to 90 seconds are immensely fit and healthy. Some yogis have a CP of 2 minutes, show highly developed intuition while being in a state of flow, and a strong ability to regenerate and heal their organism tissues.

Disease

Dr Buteyko divided the disease status into 5 categories.

Excessive breathing or hyperventilation of the lungs create a CO_2 deficiency and impede the transfer of oxygen from the blood to the cells, into the metabolism, so cellular or metabolic hypoxia occurs.

Thus, less oxygen is delivered to the body's cells and organs. When excessive breathing becomes a habit, it leads to a deterioration in metabolism and the immune system.

When reading the table, you will notice that the lower the level of CO_2 in the lungs, the more severe the stage of the disease.

Category I–IV: If the morning CP is in the range of 10 to 25 seconds, you are not healthy, you are over-breathing. The carbon dioxide level in the lungs has decreased from 6.5% (modern physiological norm) to 6.0-4.5%.

Breathing becomes deep and frequent.

Sometimes the respiratory rate increases significantly, but this fact reflects only an increase in the depth or amplitude of breathing. Increasing the depth of breathing is always primary in relation to the increase in frequency of breathing.

The homeostasis of functional systems of the organism is disturbed, so that compensatory reactions are initiated to compensate for the oxygen shortage, symptoms and diseases occur. The person has little energy, will need more sleep, has more health conditions and diseases and heavy breathing while at rest.

Category V: Dr Buteyko stated that if the morning CP is in the range of 5 seconds, the person is very ill. The CO_2 level of the lungs has dropped to 4%. The patient suffers from severe hyperventilation of the lungs, which is also noticeable in a high pulse of about 90 seconds at rest.

These figures are not exact for each patient, but reflect a trend towards an increase in the heart rate.

The homeostasis of functional systems of the organism is disturbed, compensatory mechanisms are initiated, symptoms and disease occur. The person suffers also with chronic fatigue, low self-esteem, is emotionally vulnerable and has poor memory.

The Verigo-Bohr effect

At this stage, a brief discourse on the law of physiology – the Verigo-Bohr effect – will help you understand what happens in the organism when we breathe a greater volume of air per minute than the norm, and this is the case for over 90% of modern people.

Dr Andrey Novozhilov explained to me that the Verigo-Bohr effect allows us to understand part of the healing mechanism of the Buteyko Method.

It was a Russian scientist, Bronislav Verigo from the town of Perm, who discovered in 1892 that CO_2 deficiency in the arterial blood impedes oxygen transfer from the arterial blood to the organism cells and the metabolism. The greater the deficiency of CO_2 in the arterial blood, the more difficult it is for oxygen to move from the blood to the cells. This is how cellular hypoxia occurs – a lack of oxygen in the cells, in the metabolism. In 1904, this phenomenon was repeated by Danish scientist Christian Bohr and called the Bohr effect.

Dr Andrey Novozhilov further emphasized a critical and important moment: "The exception is people with severe asthma and disturbed gas exchange in the lungs. In the arterial blood these people have very high CO_2 and low oxygen as a result of disturbed gas exchange in the destroyed lungs (emphysema and pneumo-sclerosis). So they have low CO_2 in the lungs (alveolar CO_2) and as a result a permanent bronchospasm. And they have high CO_2 and low O_2 in their arterial blood as a result of limited gas exchange in the destroyed lungs. The professors asked Buteyko why he wanted to increase CO_2 when an asthmatic has high CO_2 in the blood and dies from it? At that time, nobody understood that CO_2 could be different in the lungs and in the blood. And none of the professors at that time understood that bronchospasm is caused by low CO_2 in the lungs. Low CO_2 in the lungs is the only direct cause of bronchospasm. For this reason, the Buteyko Method can effectively treat absolutely any form of asthma."

In summary, Dr Buteyko's table shows that normal, shallow breathing is the key to good health as it normalizes gas constants in the lungs and thus normalizes the oxygen supply to the body's cells, organs and metabolism.

Deep breathing or hyperventilation leads to CO_2 deficiency in the lungs, because we exhale too much CO_2. As discovered by Dr Buteyko, deep breathing is the cause of many chronic diseases and health problems that we see in today's modern society. Every functional system, every organ and cell of the organism, the metabolism and the immune system suffer from deep breathing.

The primary aim of the Buteyko Method is therefore to reduce and normalize the respiratory volume flowing through the lungs every minute (minute volume) so that the CO_2 deficiency can be raised to a physiological norm. To reduce the volume of air, you must reduce the depth of each breath to a normal level.

Hyperventilation of the lungs: CP less than 20 seconds

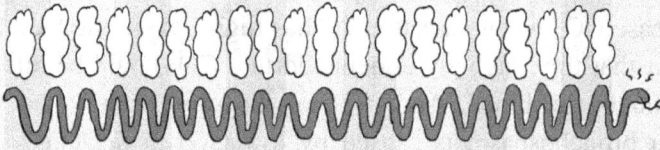

Hyperventilation of the lungs: CP of 20 to 30 seconds

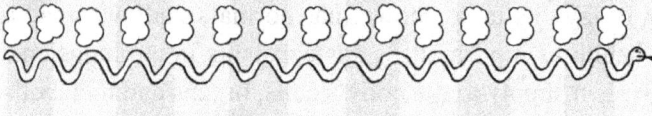

Depth of breathing (amplitude of inhalation) decreases
with increasing CP: CP of 30 to 40 seconds

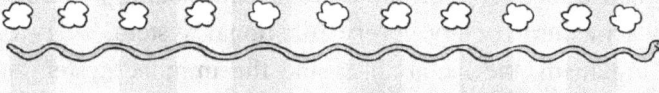

Normal shallow breathing: CP of 60 seconds

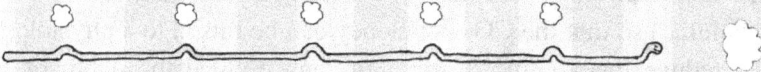

The minute volume

The minute volume

The picture of the Buteyko breathing snake illustrates in a simple way the difference between deep breathing or hyperventilation and normal shallow breathing.

The movements of the breathing snake symbolize the process of breathing, inhaling and exhaling. And the clouds above the snake symbolize the volume of air we breathe in and out.

The clouds on the right side of the picture represent the total volume of air that a person breathes in and out in one minute – the minute volume.

Hyperventilation of the lungs is carried out as a result of an increase in the depth of breathing. Without realizing it, many people breathe 2 or 3 times more volume of air in one minute than the norm. The key goal in the Buteyko Method is to heal hyperventilation by reducing, i.e. normalizing the depth of breathing.

The respiratory rate also increases with hyperventilation, but it is impossible to eliminate hyperventilation if the respiratory rate is reduced.

In the Buteyko Method we only reduce the depth of breathing, not the frequency. The frequency will reduce naturally and involuntarily, which means that the auto pause after exhalation will increase unconsciously.

Sometimes the auto pause is longer than 20 seconds and the breathing snake only takes 1-2-3 breaths per minute. This is how the amazing formula of health from Lao Tzu (2,500 years ago) is realized: "The breath of a perfect person is as if he does not breathe."

The Buteyko breathing technique is the key to returning to normal, shallow breathing by raising the morning CP above 40 seconds. What then happens is a gift: gas constants and constants of functional systems are normalized to recover and maintain good health, athletic performance and so much more.

Simple rules for normal breathing, the breathing of a healthy person

According to Dr Buteyko, the breathing of a healthy person is silent, through the nose, very gentle, slow and almost invisible.

In every situation:
- I breathe through the nose, my mouth is closed.
- I reduce the depth of breathing slightly with each inhalation, by 25% or less, without increasing the breathing rate. Dr Buteyko stated "what then occurs is a sensation of having insufficient air when the breathing is reduced".
- And pay attention to the small pause between exhaling and inhaling.

What causes hyperventilation of the lungs?

During my studies with Dr Novozhilov, I wanted to understand why most people unconsciously inhale a greater volume of air and thus deviate from a normal breathing pattern and develop symptoms or chronic disease.

There are many reasons that lead to deep breathing or hyperventilation of the lungs. One important reason which should be highlighted is the myth of deep breathing: we are often told that breathing a larger volume of air is good for us, although there is no scientific basis for this.

Furthermore, Dr Buteyko blamed the modern lifestyle: for example, the use of antibiotics, medical drugs, chronic stress, unhealthy diets, processed foods, overeating, lack of physical activity, too much sitting, too much talking, too much alcohol, tobacco, too much sleep, overheated rooms, environmental toxins and much more.

Other considerations that have a negative impact on breathing, according to Dr Buteyko, are the constant greed for more and the pleasures and addictions one craves in order to find happiness.

This does not mean one cannot drink a glass of wine or go out for dinner, dancing and so on. The Buteyko breathing technique will help you to develop a fine sense of your breathing in every situation, and you will soon find out what is good for your breathing and what is bad for your breathing. There is no need to take on stressful diets because it is impossible to normalize breathing by changing the diet, for example. Bad habits and passions will change naturally once you are really focused on increasing your morning CP to 45 seconds.

In recent years, Dr Buteyko has been increasingly saying that the main cause of excessive breathing or hyperventilation of the lungs is physical inactivity or a sedentary lifestyle.

Our physiology is arranged in such a way that we need to have strong physical activity every day for 2-4 hours. Strong physical activity, muscle work, sport are a natural mechanism for normalizing the work of the respiratory system. This is a natural mechanism for normalizing gas constants and respiratory homeostasis, but only under one condition: breathing only through the nose. The validity of this is confirmed by the fact that we have many cases of complete cure of asthma or high blood pressure through sport, but when we ask such a person about the nature of their breathing during sport, we always hear the answer that they breathed only through the nose: "My sports coach told me that if you want to stay alive with asthma and high blood pressure and doing such physical activities, then breathe only through your nose."

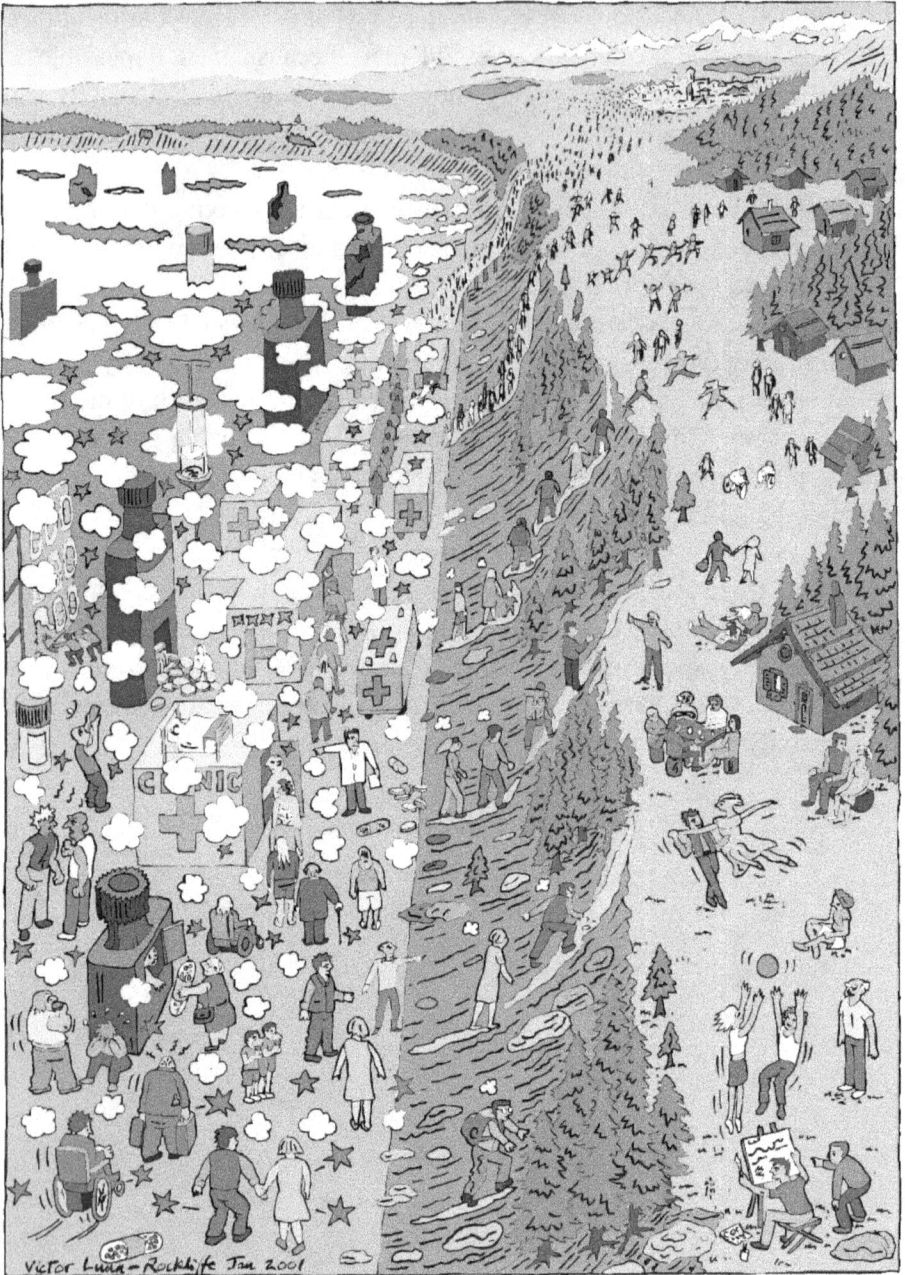

Gray dull Disease land and Green Buteyko land of Health (Buteyko Land)

Buteyko's gift to humanity from the perspective of a British artist

The British artist Victor Lunn-Rockliffe has been successfully treated using the Buteyko breathing technique (source: Butyeko's discovery from Victor Lunn-Rockliffe, 2015). The picture 'Buteyko Land' is the artist's contribution to spreading knowledge about the fundamental scientific discovery of Dr Buteyko.

The picture reflects our unhealthy modern society (see the left side of the picture). But it also shows us the way to a healthy and happy life (see the right side of the picture). Breathing is symbolized by clouds: the bigger the clouds, the more air people breathe. Looking into the future (see top left of the picture), the big clouds merge into each other. We live in a society of deep breathers, Dr Buteyko told us, and as a result our health is deteriorating and chronic diseases are rapidly increasing.

Dr Buteyko's scientific, clinical studies proved that deep breathing is the number one cause of chronic disease and suffering in today's society. A safe way to health is to learn Buteyko's breathing reduction and gradually return to normal breathing. The path is very arduous and involves hard work, but when you reach 'Buteyko Land', the reward is priceless.

Finally (bottom right of the picture), the British artist can be seen capturing the transformation of many people as they leave the modern unhealthy society and walk a new path to health, happiness and peace.

Adults and children from the age of three can learn the Buteyko breathing technique and heal chronic diseases or other health problems.

The next section is for the attention of healthy young athletes who are not so interested in hearing how to treat allergies or high blood pressure, but are very interested how to improve athletic performance using Buteyko breathing.

How the Buteyko Method improves athletic performance

Physical exercise is very important in helping to normalize your level of CO_2 and increase your CP.

The Buteyko Method helps to increase athletic endurance, athletic performance and more. The secret of this is very simple – the normalization of oxygen supply to the cells of the organism, to the metabolism.

For professional athletes it is also interesting to know that Buteyko breathing helps to avoid doping in sports, because the purpose of doping is to increase hemoglobin and this is very easy to achieve with Buteyko.

How to breathe when doing sports

Key rules are:
- Measure your CP before you start exercising.
- Breathe through your nose all the time (close your mouth).
- Maintain a slight feeling of air shortage all the time.
- Measure CP after the sport, but remember that we must measure CP under the same conditions. For example: Before the sport I was completely calm, so after the sport I have to wait for some time to completely cool down and calm down. Sometimes it takes a long time if I'm doing weightlifting.
- Or you can use another path: Take a time interval of one hour after the end of sport and measure CP every 10 minutes. After a certain interval of time, you will see that the CP begins to increase. The next time you finish a sport session, measure your CP after that time interval.
- Your CP after the exercise must be 5 seconds greater than it was before you started. If it is lower, the exercise has decreased your level of CO_2. In this case you need to reduce the intensity of your exercise to a level where you find it easier to control your breathing.

It is critical to understand that long-term breathing through the mouth is dangerous, because it is a hyperventilation of the lungs, and as a result you lose CO_2. Hyperventilation of the lungs is characterized only by CO_2 deficiency. To find out you must measure CO_2 before and after such breathing.

Athletes with morning CP above the norm

Let's look at swimming or professional boxing: these athletes breathe frequently through the mouth and deeply, but the measurement of CO_2 with the Control Pause shows high or normal CO_2 in these athletes. Why is this? Swimming or professional boxing are both power sports with a lot of physical activity that increases metabolic activity, with a lot of CO_2 production. Therefore, even with hyperventilation and mouth breathing, there is no CO_2 deficiency because we have a high CO_2 production. So, any kind of sport stimulates the metabolism and the organism always has high or normal CO_2 levels. Such athletes never get sick, despite deep breathing through the mouth.

Athletes with morning CP below the norm

Other types of athletes have the habit of breathing deeply all the time. Many athletes specifically practise the habit of deep breathing under the delusion that deep breathing provides more oxygen. This can lead to a very mild CP in the morning after a night's sleep, which indicates chronic hyperventilation and respiratory failure. The athlete compensates for the effects of hyperventilation by exercising during the day. It turns out that such an athlete has hyperventilation, weak immunity, but high CP as a result of daily physical training.

When athletes retire from sport

However, when extensive physical training ends for various reasons, usually due to the athlete's age, metabolic activity decreases, but the habit of breathing deeply through the mouth remains, and immediately there is a CO_2 deficiency and illness. This is why we see professional athletes getting sick after the end of professional physical training. The habit of breathing deeply and through the mouth kills them.

The powerful combination of Buteyko breathing and sport

Buteyko breathing studies have shown that sport in combination with deep breathing and mouth breathing cannot cure asthma or other chronic diseases and health problems.

In my personal experience, it was the powerful combination of Buteyko breathing and sport that accelerated the treatment process and full recovery of asthma. Since childhood, I have enjoyed doing a lot of sports, but the asthma could not be cured because of my excessive breathing habit. Today I know that the last thing missing was how to breathe normally, how to reduce the depth of breathing.

For some years now, Buteyko breathing has been the most important tool in my training sessions. I have increased my athletic endurance and performance since I have paid special attention to breathing normalization.

I have finally understood that normal, shallow breathing is a natural booster for health, athletic performance, personal growth, happiness and so much more. I owe my good health to the unique Russian doctor Dr Andrey Novozhilov, who passes on Buteyko's scientific heritage to people with great respect and sincerity.

In the next section you will find some useful tips for daily life to support the process of breathing normalization.

Buteyko for daily life

How to breathe during a night's sleep

Take a look at your sleeping habits: Do you sleep on your back, sleep with your mouth open, snore, wake up at night or in the morning with a dry mouth or blocked nose? These are clear signs of excessive breathing and hyperventilation.

Sleeping on the stomach is important for people who suffer from hyperventilation at night. This position naturally reduces the depth of breathing due to the gentle pressure of your organism's weight on the diaphragm. Another good position is the side position, with either both knees or one knee bent.

Measure your CP before going to sleep. Then measure your CP in the morning after waking – it should be 5 seconds higher than the night before. If not, you are breathing too much while you sleep. A low CP also means that you are sleeping too many hours. If your morning CP is higher than the night before, you have better sleep, no hyperventilation, and you feel fitter.

It can be very helpful to set yourself an alarm clock that wakes you every two or three hours. Measure your CP every time you wake. Try to do breathing exercises when you have symptoms. This helps to avoid an asthma attack.

You may want to put a medical tape vertically on your mouth to remind you to close your mouth while sleeping.

Coughing

Try to pay attention to how you cough. Do you cough with an open mouth? Maybe you use extra force to clear the mucus from the bronchial tubes?

The main danger of coughing is a sudden forced expiration which causes a significant CO_2 loss in the lungs. Coughing is a common cause of hyperventilation, as almost everyone takes a deep breath after coughing. Coughing can also be a symptom, for example, of flu.

The recommendation is to cough not at all, or at least with a closed mouth to avoid hyperventilation and the loss of vital CO_2 in the lungs. This is because hyperventilation constricts the bronchial tubes, changes the viscosity of the mucus and prevents the natural discharge of mucus. To prevent microbial infection, mucus clearance should be normalized, and to do this, the hyperventilation of the lungs must first be eliminated.

With the help of Buteyko breathing exercises, the CO_2 level in the lungs will increase and mucus can be cleared effortlessly. After every cough (coughing is exhalation), simply block your nose with the fingers and hold the breath for three to five seconds, which will prevent an increase of CO_2 loss as a result of coughing. You can add the relaxation exercise.

Sneezing

It doesn't really matter whether you sneeze with your mouth open or closed, because sneezing is much less common than coughing and therefore rarely provokes an asthma attack.

Another important thing: sneezing is a sharp forced expiration as when coughing, and also leads to a loss of CO_2; therefore, after each sneeze, you need to stop breathing for 3 to 5 seconds to compensate for the loss of CO_2.

After every sneeze, block your nose with the fingers and hold your breath for a few seconds to compensate for the loss of CO_2 due to the forced exhalation. After the breath hold, you can wipe your nose. Try to avoid wiping the nose before the breath hold, because it is followed by a deep inhalation.

Clearing a blocked nose

Many people suffer from chronic rhinitis or blocked nose. The cause is excessive CO_2 loss in the lungs due to hyperventilation.

To compensate for the CO_2 loss: after a normal exhalation, block the nose with your fingers and hold the breath for five seconds. After holding your breath, you can blow your nose gently without breathing.

Alternatively: After a normal exhalation, hold the breath with a medium to strong effort of willpower and start walking, running or jumping. When you start breathing again, pay attention to the depth of the first breath; the inhalation should not be increased, but you can easily control the breathing and (with an effort of willpower) reduce the increased depth of breathing to normal. Relax for 30 to 60 seconds and repeat until symptoms have disappeared.

Stopping headaches

Many people suffer from headaches. With a headache, there is always hyperventilation of the lungs, which is easy to find out if you measure the CP.

To relieve a headache, try reducing the depth of your breathing through relaxation.

Start relaxing the facial muscles, relax the forehead, relax the muscles around the eyes to stop blinking with muscle relaxation, relax the lower jaw so that it is not compressed.

It is enough to relax the muscles of the face, back of the head and neck to eliminate the headache and feel the automatic decrease in the depth of breathing.

Please note that the headache will go away only when the depth of breathing is automatically reduced; the easiest way to get this effect is to relax the muscles whose tone affects the depth of breathing.

To stop the headache, relax your breathing muscles until the symptoms are gone.

Breath holds for busy people

If you do not have the motivation and discipline to practise Buteyko breathing exercises, then make a lot of breath holds during the day:
After a normal exhalation, block your nose and hold your breath comfortably for 1 second, or 2 seconds, or 3 seconds, then continue normal breathing. Repeat 400 to 500 times a day, at university, online lectures, work, cinema, shopping, cooking and so on.

Historical excursion: How breathing exercises based on deep breathing and hyperventilation of the lungs appeared

In the early 19th century, according to Dr Andrey Novozhilov, the French scientist and physician, René Laennec, first suspected the existence of bronchospasm in patients with bronchial asthma.

Following elementary logic, he suggested that a narrowing of the bronchi is the reason for the insufficient functioning of the respiratory function. Laennec concluded that the air input through the narrowed bronchi should be increased in order to normalize the respiratory function. Thus began the era of breathing exercises based on deep breathing.

His mistake was that he did not measure the respiration function parameters, so he could not see that lung ventilation in patients with asthma significantly exceeded the norm.

Surprisingly, until the end of the 20th century and before Buteyko's scientific research, no scientists thought to measure the parameters of respiratory function in patients with asthma, but everyone continued to recommend deep breathing to such patients.

Here is an analogy: The science of astronomy says that the Earth revolves around the Sun. But every day I see a completely different thing: The Sun rises in the East and sets in the West, therefore, the Sun rotates around the Earth.

Who is right? Only scientific measurements provide the correct answer to this question.

It is the same situation with the Buteyko Method: Doctors say that patients with asthma have narrowed bronchi, therefore the respiratory function does not work enough or normally.

But scientific measurements of respiratory function parameters show that lung ventilation is above normal, therefore the function is excessive.

In this case, we must look at the narrowing of the bronchi as a special mechanism, the work of which prevents the flow of excess air.

To get an answer to the question about the quality of work of any functional system of the organism, we must first look at the indicators of physiological parameters, look at the indicators of constant values that are supported by the work of this functional system.

If the indicators of the constants that the operation of this functional system supports are normal, we say that the system is working normally.

If the indicators of the constants are changed, increased or decreased, then we say that this functional system works insufficiently or excessively, depending on what it should do - increase or decrease the constant.

For example, if we see a lack of thyroid hormone, then we say that the work of this endocrine system is disrupted and the system does not work enough.

If we see CO_2 deficiency in the lungs, then we say that the work of the external respiration system (lung ventilation) is excessive, because the CO_2 constant is lowered.

The CO_2 constant is critical because it regulates the supply of oxygen to the metabolism, and with the development of CO_2 deficiency, the organism will die; but first compensatory reactions (the so-called homeostatic reactions) will occur, the work of which will tend to normalize the CO_2 constant in the lungs. This is bronchospasm and reversible bronchial obstruction with the outcome in pneumofibrosis (destruction of the lungs), which will gradually occur if the CO2 constant in the lungs normalizes very slowly or does not normalize at all.

Therefore, as Dr Buteyko says, I wish you good health with normal, shallow breathing!

My true path of learning, practising and teaching the Buteyko breathing technique

Claudia Schyia

Certified Buteyko Method specialist

Cologne, Germany

"To develop good health and new thinking, one needs to breathe less, eat less, sleep less and physically work harder to the point of sweating one's brow. Hyperventilation is the cause of oxygen deficiency which also affects the cerebral cortex. When the cerebral cortex falls asleep due to lack of oxygen, the subcortical instincts take over, which is to eat and reproduce, aggression etc. We are turning into animals. This is what we see around us in today's culture and civilisation."

Dr Konstantin P. Buteyko, MD, PhD, author of the Buteyko Method

Only now do I truly understand the quote from Dr Buteyko. For me, learning the Buteyko breathing technique (BBT) from the Moscow Classic School has been the greatest gift of my life, although it has also been the most difficult path I have ever walked. The experience of practising BBT with patience and zeal has healed my chronic asthma, my perception and way of thinking, as if a light has come into my cerebral cortex. BBT is a life-changing practice as it also normalizes the oxygen flow in the cerebral cortex, leading to conscious living and mental and spiritual growth.

I would like to draw the attention of the reader to the Classic Buteyko School in Moscow, the only source of genuine true knowledge about the patented Buteyko Method. The Buteyko Method can be applied by a medical doctor or a specially trained Buteyko specialist with annual certification from the Moscow Classic School. I am sincerely grateful to the master of the classic Buteyko Method, Dr Andrey Novozhilov, for his excellent teaching, his wise guidance and continued mentoring and support.

Simply start to discover the great simplicity of the Buteyko Method

Online Buteyko studies include both treatment for patients and training to be a qualified Buteyko practitioner. No special knowledge is required to participate in the Buteyko classes. The beginner is not given a script; it is about listening and concentrating on the breath. Without a doubt, the Buteyko breath study is the most valuable study I have experienced in my entire life. Not only have I been cured of chronic asthma disease, but I have also increased my physical and mental fitness. It feels like being new born, and most importantly, it has changed my life to follow the inner path, unite with my breath and recognize my true self.

The value of the Buteyko Method is infinite. It has shown me the way to awaken and develop my attention span to the point of perfect concentration and consciousness that shapes the invisible part of my being. Being in the state of Buteyko breathing is like a silent path of love through the rush and hypocrisy of modern life.

I am often asked why I have not consulted a German Buteyko teacher, and the answer is simple. As an asthma patient for over four decades, I have become very critical of doctors and have lost confidence as they only treat the symptoms but not the cause of the chronic disease. Unfortunately, the German and Western world is flooded with non-genuine Buteyko teachers who neither have an annual certification from the Moscow Classic School nor an official licence to teach the patented Buteyko Method.

The importance of a master guiding the beginner

Without the guidance of a genuine master, the beginner cannot be successful.

I remember the very first lesson with Dr Novozhilov and his prompt diagnosis: "The cause of your asthma is your excessive breathing. Once you normalize your breathing pattern, you will be free of asthma." Was it that simple? For over 40 years German doctors told me the opposite, that chronic asthma cannot be cured.

My motivation was truly strengthened, even though it meant pursuing a very challenging goal: two hours of daily Buteyko practice were necessary to achieve a morning CP of 45 seconds.

Morning CP development

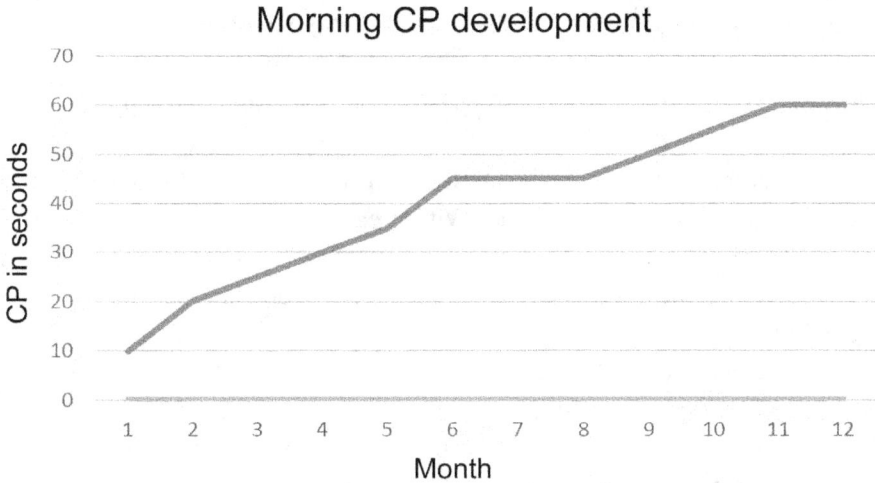

My difficult journey to normalize breathing

At the beginning of my practice, the morning CP was 10 seconds; and after exactly six months of practice I achieved a morning CP of 45 seconds. According to the Moscow School, adults need 3 to 6 months and children 4 weeks. I still remember the happy day, and especially my first thought that now that I had reached the goal, I could rest and stop practising every day.

My symptoms have completely disappeared; I no longer take medication and have gained enormous energy and good health.

But the Moscow Classic School set a second goal for me: to maintain the morning CP of 45 seconds for the next 6 months and beyond.

My difficult journey to normalize my breathing continued with daily practice. It is not an easy task to sit alone in silence, trying to put all thoughts aside, be calm and patient and concentrate on breathing reduction. It requires a lot of discipline and an attentive mind.

In my personal experience, the beginner feels initial difficulties due to our modern education, because we have never learned to spend dedicated time with ourselves in absolute silence without distraction and just focus on breathing. Instead, from an early age, we are trapped on a hamster wheel where we learn to run faster and breathe deeper in order to adapt to the world around us. We are not aware of the danger of deep breathing and the power of normal breathing, the reduction of the depth of breathing.

The turning point in my difficult Buteyko journey

Next to dedicated breathing practice, a burning desire and thirst for more Buteyko knowledge awoke in me. With great enthusiasm and support from the Moscow Classic School, the first manuscript was completed to deepen my physiological, theoretical and practical understanding of Buteyko breathing.

Completely unexpectedly, after more than a year of daily Buteyko practice, I have noticed a turning point where practising has become a loving devotion. I no longer have to force myself as I used to. It no longer feels difficult, but has become easy and likable, so that as soon as I stop daily practice, I feel a need to continue. Especially during sport, I have successfully cultivated nasal breathing and also kept up a slight feeling of lack of air. I cannot imagine breathing through my mouth any more, not even during high-intensity training. As a result, my performance has significantly improved and I enjoy physical activities even more.

Now, after more than 3 years of diligent practice, my morning CP is almost 60 seconds. I feel immensely fit and am free of viral and other infections. However, the most magical morning CP I ever experienced was

2 minutes. My breathing muscles were automatically relaxing one after the other, generating a lightness all over my body and a peaceful state of mind.

According to the Moscow Classic School, the next level of Buteyko breathing normalization is to develop a consciousness of breathing, to feel and control my breathing when I am doing sport, when I am talking to people: at all times, whatever I am doing. I have noticed that I think a lot about my breathing pattern, as if my organism is trying to remind me to pay attention to breathe a lower volume of air in every situation.

It is a great honour to be part of the real Buteyko family, to have experienced a new way of learning – without PowerPoint presentations or handouts – simply by concentrating on breathing reduction. Without the professional guidance of Dr Novozhilov, a unique physician and wise master of the classic Buteyko Method, I would not have been able to achieve such good results.

It is also a special privilege to hold the annual certificate of the Moscow Classic School. As an official representative of the Moscow Classic School, I am authorized to give Buteyko breathing courses.

Teaching Buteyko breathing at the University sports programme

Despite my severe respiratory illness, I studied sport at the University of Munich and the German Sport University Cologne (GSUC) and graduated in 1991 with a Master's degree in Sports Science.

For more than 30 years, I have been teaching fitness courses at the Cologne University sports programme. Dr Andrey Novozhilov encouraged me to also teach Buteyko breathing courses. Thus, I spent many months preparing a teaching manuscript under constant supervision and guidance from Moscow. Since the winter semester of 2020, I have been teaching Buteyko breathing courses. The course is dedicated to Professor Konstantin Buteyko (1923–2003) and Dr Andrey Novozhilov, out of deepest gratitude.

How to become a successful Buteyko teacher

"To be a successful Buteyko practitioner, you will also teach the Buteyko breathing technique (BBT) a little differently, not the way I taught you," stated Dr Novozhilov.

You must remember

BBT normalizes the respiratory function and therefore can be used in all situations (there are no absolute contra-indications).

BBT is based on the principle of gradually reducing the depth of breathing to normal, which can be done in very different ways: by delaying breathing after exhalation, by muscle relaxation, the tone of which affects the depth of breathing, and finally by physical activity/sport when breathing only through the nose.

Working with other people will help you to reduce the depth of breathing properly. Professor Buteyko said, learn from your patients how to reduce the depth of breathing.

"Doctor, before you cure your patients, you have to cure yourself," said Professor Buteyko. Every Buteyko practitioner or doctor should have a CP of 40 seconds; and, most importantly, when you conduct Buteyko classes with patients, you must correctly reduce the depth of breathing yourself. The professor called this 'skill in golden words': to be a little bit in the Buteyko Method, you should be able to create a pleasant, comfortable lack of air and keep yourself in this state.

Patients almost always use the same method you use to reduce breathing, because it is intuitively very easy to feel during Buteyko practice. If it is pleasant and comfortable for you to reduce the depth of breathing, it will also be pleasant and comfortable for your patients to reduce their breathing, and they will quickly experience an improvement in their condition.

Teaching Buteyko breathing is the greatest enrichment of my life. I have been inspired by Anna's excellent teaching skills: the Buteyko online courses in the summer of 2021 with Anna and Laura have helped me to develop my own teaching style. Anna inherited the special gift of teaching the Buteyko breathing technique from her father, Dr Andrey Novozhilov, and her grandmother, Dr Lyudmila Buteyko (Novozhilova).

Teaching experience with Buteyko beginners

The Buteyko breathing course is recommended for all students to improve their athletic performance and strengthen their respiratory, immune/ metabolic and nervous systems, blood circulation and general health. Interestingly, no student has a morning CP of 40 to 45 seconds. Most are in the range of 20 to 30 seconds. Teaching others also has a positive impact on my own Buteyko breathing performance: it helps me on my way to attain breathing perfection.

I still remember the very first Buteyko class. After the class a biology student approached me and emphasized his great interest in breathing. He told me about his negative experiences in other breathing courses, where participants were encouraged to breathe in deeply and to exhale through the mouth, which made him feel dizzy. He was also very interested in the Verigo-Bohr effect, especially the Russian scientist Bronislav Verigo. It is inspiring and motivating to meet young people who are interested in Buteyko breathing, which is the opposite of the Western mantra of deep breathing.

"Remember the Christian story, when the apostle Paul spoke in the Areopagus about resurrection after death and eternal life; many laughed and listened incredulously. But after his speech there were two people who approached him and began to listen very carefully to his story. One of them was the great Dionysius the Areopagite. There will always be followers and people who are interested," said Dr Novozhilov.

I have to admit that I did not remember the apostle Paul, but I felt an urgent need to find out. At that particular moment I discovered a love of reading the Gospels and the lives of the Saints. The apostle Paul spoke the truth about Christ as the long-promised Messiah and Saviour of the world. Saint Dionysius the Areopagite was baptised by Saint Paul in Athens and is one of the seventy apostles chosen by the Lord.

My personal experience has shown that "there will always be followers and people who are interested". Almost every week new students join the

Buteyko class: some come back, who are curious and open to learn; others are not. Sometimes students come with yoga mats and are disappointed when I explain that it is not a yoga breathing class. However, a core group of students attend every weekly session. We often practice in two groups: beginners and advanced. It is amazing how the spirit of 'being a bit in the Buteyko Method' magically transfers to others, whether they are beginners or advanced. A funny moment occurs when students stop controlling their depth of breathing and return to their usual breathing. You can see great relief in their happy faces.

Most students are physically fit and find it easy to implement the breathing instructions immediately. They prefer Buteyko breathing while walking or running, as it is easier to reduce the depth of breathing than while sitting.

The students are also very grateful for tips for everyday life: for example, breathing during sleep, dealing with hyperventilation during a night's rest, how to stop coughing, sneezing, how to clear a blocked nose, stop headaches.

At the end of the course, participants share their daily experiences with Buteyko breathing. For example, one student experienced: "During sports, especially endurance sports, I notice that I am much more efficient and have more endurance when I only breathe in and out through my nose. I really recommend it. My morning CP has improved from 20 seconds to 33 seconds. My only mistake is not practising in a disciplined manner. The exercises themselves are child's play."

Let's make a brief excursion to yoga and Christianity and the analogy to Buteyko breathing

Dr Buteyko deciphered the secret of breathing and longevity of yogis, the secret of the fortitude of ancient Christian ascetics and made this knowledge available to people.

Most yoga teachers would say that it is important to breathe deeply to get more oxygen into the body. It seems that the true teachings of yoga have been distorted from their original power and meaning when taught by many modern practitioners. If you look up the ancient Sanskrit literature of yoga, nowhere is it written that deep breathing leads to greater health, but it does emphasize breathing reduction and controlled breathing.

It is important to understand that the breathing of yogis is not hyperventilation of the lungs, especially when we talk about the so-called full breathing of yogis.

Why isn't this hyperventilation?

The technique of full yogi breathing looks very simple, but it is impossible to do it without a master.

When doing the full breathing of the yogis, one should make only one inhalation and one exhalation per minute. This is the technique of full slow breathing of the yogis and it cannot be done without special training with a master.

The secret of why the yogis' full breathing normalizes the work of the respiratory system is also very simple. During the deepest slowest inhalation, we can physically (technically) inhale only 5 litres of air and exhale the same amount during the fullest slowest exhalation. The lung capacity of an adult is about 5 litres.

We know that the ventilation of the lungs of a healthy person is 5 litres of air per minute, and we unwittingly get this result during such a special breathing technique. The difficulty of the full breathing of yogis lies in performing only one inhalation and exhalation per minute, and the secret to normalizing the work of the respiratory system is contained in one word: slow.

It is also astonishing that in the world's practised religions, and primarily in Christianity, the Holy fathers of the Church indicate: hold your breath during prayer, do not breathe boldly, connect prayer and breathing. This has been forgotten today.

The spiritual development of the personality is always connected with breathing.

For example, John of the Ladder in his book *Ladder* writes: "Let the memory about Jesus unite with your breath; then you will know the benefits of silence."

Very impressing are also the words of the 7th-century Christian ascetic Isaac the Syrian, who said that "Silence (silentness, free of passion) is the secret of the coming century, and words are the instrument of the present century."

Silence (silentness) here implies not only the absence of words or speech, but also silence as a special state of mind (soul) that has been given freedom from passions.

Here an interesting analogy arises with the Buteyko Method: we know that a decrease in breathing according to Buteyko (what we call 'being a bit in the Buteyko Method' or 'light comfortable breathlessness according to Buteyko') has several properties:

- it concentrates your attention,
- makes you silent,
- and involuntarily, as Professor Buteyko said, regardless of our desire, it reduces passion (reduces the effect of the passions on us).

It turns out that the reduction of breathing according to Buteyko frees one from the passions. In other words, 'being a bit in the Buteyko Method' is a mechanism, or a way, or a technique that brings us closer to silence (silentness), frees us from the passions and brings us closer to the mystery of the coming century.

It turns out that the Buteyko Method, the Buteyko breathing technique, is the medicine of the next century, and antibiotics and steroids are the instrument of medicine of the present century.

Concentration of attention

Decreasing the depth of breathing is a natural mechanism for concentrating attention, forming and developing awareness. Many people use the buzzword 'mindfulness', but no one explains what it is.

Mindfulness (awareness) is the concentration of attention that arises when the depth of breathing is reduced, according to Buteyko.

In the Buteyko Method there are natural ways to normalize the work of the breathing system and to reduce the depth of breathing (these are correct posture and relaxation). In the same way to form the skill of concentration, a natural mechanism should be used in order to create a slight decrease in the depth of breathing.

Undoubtedly, when thinking about something important or simply interesting, many people have paid attention to holding their breath at these moments, to an involuntary (unconscious, automatic) decrease in the depth of breathing, or to an involuntary but short-term cessation (stop) of breathing for some seconds.

It is also important to note that Christian ascetic literature is full of a search for ways to concentrate attention during prayer, and today we know that a slight decrease in the depth of breathing according to Buteyko can be used as a natural mechanism to concentrate attention.

At the same time, both Christian asceticism and Dr Buteyko constantly point out that unreasonable interference in the breathing process leads to madness.

Unreasonable interference in the breathing process leads to madness, why?

Because there are laws of physiology, the violation of which leads to illness, madness and death. Dr Buteyko gave us the 'correct', scientifically grounded and for this reason absolutely safe way to work with breathing, based on knowledge and study of the laws of physiology.

However, the Buteyko technique will be safe and effective only in the hands of a specialist who has an annual certificate from the Buteyko Clinic in Moscow.

Dr Buteyko's scientific discovery is as fundamental to humanity as the development of antibiotics to treat an infection or steroids to treat asthma, while the use of the Buteyko Method exceeds the effect of steroids in the treatment of asthma.

Finally, I would like to express my deepest gratitude to the Buteyko Clinic in Moscow for preserving the original, genuine Buteyko Method that Dr Konstantin Buteyko taught people. You have enriched my life enormously. May God bless you.

Epilogue by Dr Andrey E. Novozhilov

Dr Andrey E. Novozhilov, MD

co-author of the Buteyko Method, copyright holder (since 2014)

co-founder and chief physician of the Buteyko Clinic in Moscow (est. 1987)

The ability to control breathing within a wide framework, given to us by nature, creates the illusion of permissiveness and a kind of impunity when performing actions with breathing, but this is far from the real case.

Once a patient from Germany came to me to the Buteyko Clinic in Moscow who for many years had suffered from a severe form of bronchial asthma, which he had decided to try to fight with the help of yogi breathing.

It is well known that the breathing of yogis often has a positive effect in the treatment of this disease, and not finding a good teacher he had decided to study the so-called yogi breathing by himself from the available literature. A day later he had ended up in the hospital emergency ward with a severe attack of suffocation.

When I asked him to show me what he was doing from the available literature, he showed me the monstrous deep breathing and hyperventilation of the lungs at a very fast pace.

I then asked him if he knew the correct name for this famous yoga technique - very deep and very slow breathing?

"No," he replied, "in the description of this breathing technique of yogis the word 'slow' was absent."

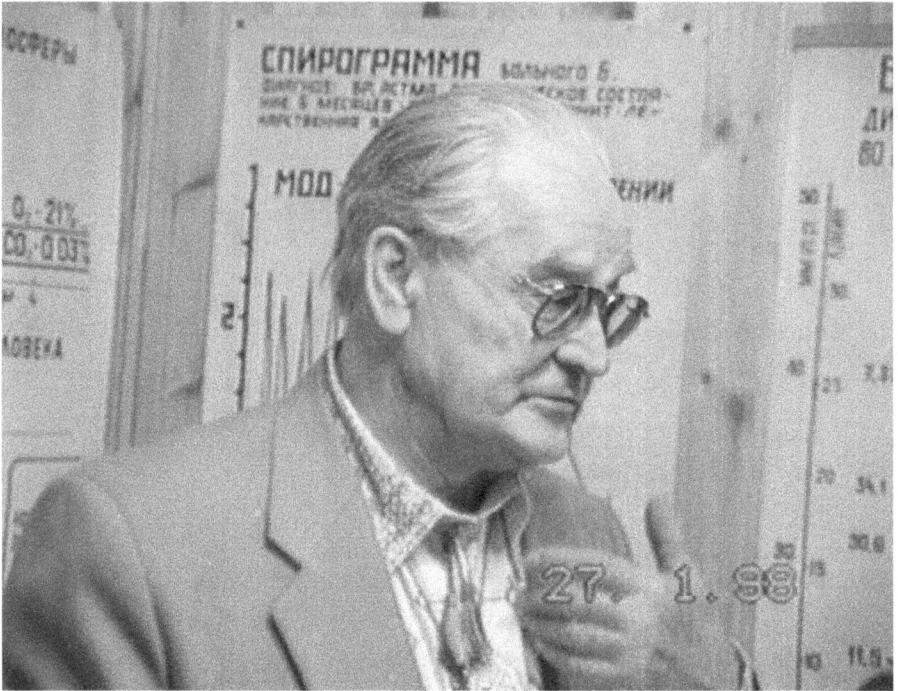

Dr Konstantin P. Buteyko, 1998

For some reason, the interpreters of the available literature on the breathing of yogis missed only one word in their description of the famous yogi technique, and it was the absence of this one word that almost led the patient with asthma to death.

Here you have an example of an unreasonable approach to manipulations of breathing and what they may lead to.

Dr Buteyko, as a doctor and scientist, was the first in medicine to approach breathing control from a scientific point of view. He studied the key parameters that change during volitional control of breathing and pointed out the CO_2 constant, which must be measured before and after performing any manipulations with breathing to assess the effectiveness of treatment.

A review of the literature and information available in the world about the Buteyko Method shows that today the only source of genuine, true knowledge about Dr Buteyko and the Buteyko Method is the Moscow Clinic, founded by the author Dr Konstantin P. Buteyko, and the two co-authors Dr Lyudmila D. Buteyko (Novozhilova) and Dr Andrey E. Novozhilov.

We have more than 40 years of personal and professional communication experience with Dr Buteyko; we hold the scientific archive of Dr Buteyko, with its bank of video recordings of lectures, seminars for patients and specialists conducted by Dr Konstantin Buteyko and Dr Lyudmila Buteyko (Novozhilova).

In terms of knowledge and scientific information, this archive has no equal in the world.

We use all this unique knowledge to treat patients effectively and train new specialists.

Today there is a lot of fake and simply false information about the Buteyko Method, and I often talk about it in videos on our YouTube channel.

Be very careful when accessing sources of information about the Buteyko Method. Please contact only specialists who are certified by the Buteyko Clinic in Moscow (est. 1987) and have a Specialist Certificate that contains the logo and signature of the copyright holder and has a validity period of one year.

Be attentive to your breathing and, as Dr Buteyko said, I wish you health and happiness from no deep breathing!

Warm wishes,

Dr Andrey E. Novozhilov, MD

Glossary of Buteyko Method terms, with explanations by Dr Andrey E. Novozhilov

Dr Andrey E. Novozhilov, MD

co-author of the Buteyko Method, copyright holder (since 2014)

co-founder and chief physician of the Buteyko Clinic in Moscow (est. 1987)

For the first time in practice, we give a scientific definition of the terms that are used when describing the Buteyko Method, such as the 'Buteyko Method', 'deep breathing', 'The art of reducing the depth of breathing with a light volitional effort' or 'The art of ephemeral, imperceptible breathing' and many others.

We will be glad to correct any discrepancies or ambiguities if readers are uncertain of any meanings.

The terms are presented in alphabetical order.

The terms presented in *italics* come from the text, and are given an explanation.

Alveolar hyperventilation

(hyperventilation of the lungs, deep breathing)

This is an increase in ventilation of the pulmonary alveoli which are in contact with blood in the gas exchange zone, with unchanged or reduced metabolic activity.

It is the cause of alveolar hypocapnia, respiratory homeostasis disorders and deep breathing disease.

Dr K. Buteyko identified prolonged inactivity with a subsequent decrease in metabolic activity, as well as *deep breathing* with unchanged metabolic activity, as the reasons.

Alveolar hypocapnia

A reduction of the partial pressure of carbon dioxide *(pCO$_2$)* in the alveolar air of the lungs.

The main causes are prolonged inactivity (*hypodynamia*) and *alveolar hyperventilation (hyperventilation of the lungs, deep breathing)*.

It is the cause of the formation of *homeostatic reactions of the functional respiratory system,* the clinical manifestation of which are *reversible bronchial obstruction, bronchospasm, peripheral angiospasm* and increased blood pressure.

In diseases with impaired diffusion of respiratory gases through the alveolo-capillary membrane (pneumofibrosis), alveolar hypocapnia can occur simultaneously with *arterial hypercapnia* (excess CO$_2$ in arterial blood). It often leads to the patient's death.

In the treatment of bronchial asthma with *arterial hypercapnia*, the breathing techniques of *the Buteyko Method* normalize the CO$_2$ *constant* in the lungs and eliminate *bronchospasm*, which makes it possible to restore gas exchange through intact areas of the lungs and remove excess CO$_2$ from the blood.

Elimination of *hyperventilation of the lungs* using *the Buteyko Method* allows the removal of excess CO$_2$ from arterial blood.

Dr K. Buteyko emphasized that the main cause of alveolar hypocapnia is a sedentary lifestyle, inactivity, *hypodynamia*, which leads to a decrease in metabolic activity and *deep breathing*.

As a preventive measure, Dr K. Buteyko pointed out the need for muscular (physical) activity for at least two hours a day, which allows normalizing the activity of metabolism and the *constant* CO_2.

Apnea

From the ancient Greek - absence of breathing, stopping of breathing.

Arterial hypocapnia and arterial hypertension

A reduction of carbon dioxide *(pCO₂)* in arterial blood due to *hyperventilation of the lungs, deep breathing* and prolonged inactivity *(hypodynamia)*.

Arterial hypertension

Increased blood pressure due to a decrease in carbon dioxide *(pCO₂)* in arterial blood and spasm of blood vessels *(peripheral angiospasm)*.

The scientific research of Dr K. Buteyko and his students demonstrated the relationship between *hyperventilation of the lungs*, prolonged inactivity *(hypodynamia)* and *peripheral angiospasm* with increased blood pressure.

In accordance with the theory of *deep breathing disease* proposed by the Russian physiologist and physician Dr K. Buteyko, *metabolic hypoxia* appears due to *deep breathing* (a deficiency of CO_2 in arterial blood, according to *the Verigo-Bohr effect*, makes it difficult for oxygen to pass from the blood into the cells).

To eliminate metabolic hypoxia, peripheral angiospasm occurs, the physiological meaning of which is to increase blood pressure in order to increase the speed and volume of blood flow per unit of time through a unit area.

Peripheral angiospasm and arterial hypertension, which have arisen in order to eliminate *metabolic hypoxia*, are functional (reversible) homeostatic reactions, the low efficiency of which will cause an increase in cholesterol and the development of atherosclerosis of blood vessels, which should be considered as organic (irreversible) homeostatic reactions of the physiological *functional respiratory system.*

The medical technology created by Dr K. Buteyko, known as *the Buteyko Method*, makes it possible to cure without drugs those diseases that occur with an increase in blood pressure, an increase in cholesterol and the development of atherosclerosis of blood vessels.

Arterial hypercapnia

An increase of carbon dioxide (CO_2) in arterial blood.

It can occur in patients with bronchial asthma as a result of a decrease in the area of gas exchange in the lungs and ineffective removal of CO_2 during respiration (prolonged *bronchospasm* and functional blood bypass).

It also occurs with extensive pneumofibrosis as a result of impaired diffusion of respiratory gases through the alveoli-capillary membrane, as a result of which venous blood with a high content of CO_2 enters the arterial bed (organic blood bypass).

Dr K. Buteyko pointed out that for the treatment of diseases with arterial hypercapnia, it is necessary to normalize air access to intact areas of the lungs, which will remove excess CO_2 from the blood.

For example, for the treatment of severe bronchial asthma occurring with hypercapnia, it is necessary first of all to eliminate hyperventilation of the lungs and normalize the CO_2 constant in the lungs in order to eliminate bronchial obstruction, bronchospasm and remove excess CO_2 through intact areas of the lungs.

The practice of treating patients with Covid-19 has shown the following: 20% of the normal, usual area of gas exchange is sufficient to ensure normal arterial blood saturation (93-98%) and normal CO_2 removal in the absence of *bronchospasm* and *bronchial obstruction.*

Breathing

The exchange of gases between the atmosphere and the cells of the organism.

In the process of evolution, environmental conditions were changing and *physiological functional systems* were formed that ensured the maintenance of *constants* within the normal range.

For example, a complex *functional respiratory system* has been formed to maintain such vital *constants* as oxygen (O_2) and carbon dioxide (CO_2) in the cell.

At first, respiration was carried out by simple diffusion of gases through the shell of a single-celled organism.

With the formation of multicellular organisms, it became necessary to transfer gases from the surface layers of the organism to the internal areas. In particular, for this purpose, the blood and circulatory system was formed as a transport site of *the functional respiratory system*.

And only later, as the structures and functions of the organism became more complicated, a *functional system* of external respiration was formed, providing ventilation of the alveoli of the lungs in contact with blood.

The ultimate goal of the entire respiratory system is to maintain O_2 and CO_2 in cells and tissues at a normal level.

Respiratory homeostasis is the constancy of the gas composition of blood and tissues. (Dr K. Buteyko, 'Regulation of bronchial tone in healthy people and patients with bronchial asthma'. Institute of Physiology of the Siberian Branch of the USSR Academy of Sciences, Novosibirsk, Akademgorodok, 1967, manuscript)

Buteyko breathing exercises

The descriptions of the Buteyko breathing techniques in the Glossary are presented for general reference. Please contact a specialist who is certified by the Buteyko Clinic in Moscow (est. 1987) to perform the Buteyko breathing exercises correctly. Please make sure the specialist's certificate has a logo, the signature of the copyright holder and a validity period of one year.

Buteyko breathing exercises are part of a non-medicinal method of treatment known as the Buteyko Method.

Three ways for the Buteyko Method's treatment and recovery

1. Buteyko breathing exercises for the normalization of gas constants and respiratory homeostasis through the elimination of excessive breathing.
2. Dosed physical (muscular) activity (under the control of the dynamics of pulmonary ventilation) to normalize gas constants and respiratory homeostasis by increasing the activity of metabolism.
3. Search, analysis and elimination of the causes of excessive breathing for the prevention of respiratory homeostasis disorders.

Buteyko breathing exercises allow patients to normalize gas constants at all levels of activity of the physiological functional system of respiration: in the lungs (the so-called functional system of external respiration), in the blood (the transport system for respiratory gases), in the cells (the level of metabolism).

Normalization of respiratory homeostasis makes it possible to cancel the action of compensatory (homeostatic) reactions of the functional respiratory system, the essence of which is the normalization of gas constants and respiratory homeostasis.

Normalization of respiratory homeostasis makes it possible to eliminate the clinical manifestations of these homeostatic reactions: to eliminate chronic nasal congestion, eliminate reversible bronchial obstruction, normalize cholesterol and high blood pressure, and a number of other treatments without medication.

Some types of Buteyko breathing exercises

1. Natural methods to eliminate excessive ventilation of the lungs by relaxing and by correcting posture.
2. Volitional methods to eliminate excessive ventilation of the lungs with the help of volitional reduction of breathing depth or volitional breath holdings.
3. A combination of natural and volitional ways of breathing normalizations.
4. A combination of natural and volitional methods of breathing normalizations in combination with dosed physical (muscular) activity under the control of the dynamics of pulmonary ventilation.

Some special terms in the Buteyko breathing exercises

Deep breathing reduction, decrease breathing volume, reduction of respiration, reduced breathing (according to Dr K. Buteyko)

A special term in *the Buteyko breathing exercises or the Buteyko Method* to denote one of the ways to normalize the functioning of the physiological *functional respiratory system*, which is based on the principle of *the Buteyko Method - a gradual decrease of the depth of breathing to normal*.

Dr K. Buteyko's scientific research has shown that it is precisely the decrease in the depth of respiration that makes it possible to normalize *gas constants* at all levels of the *functional respiratory system* - in the lungs, in the blood, in the cells.

Changing other parameters of the breathing pattern does not effectively normalize *respiratory homeostasis*.

See the description of the Buteyko breathing exercise 'Volitional liquidation of deep breathing' or 'The art of ephemeral, imperceptible breathing' or the exercise 'Pleasant air shortage or slight hunger for air'.

Breathlessness (in relation to the Buteyko breathing exercises)

A visual characteristic of the unique state of the function of external respiration or pulmonary ventilation, in which breathing is literally 'not visible and not audible'. It is one of the Buteyko breathing exercises based on a natural way to normalize gas constants and work of the respiratory system.

It is one of the key indicators of *health* and is characteristic of a healthy person at rest.

It also occurs when performing some breathing techniques of the Buteyko Method, when there is an automatic decrease in the depth of breathing as a result of consistent relaxation and correct posture, which is accompanied by a feeling of 'comfort that one does not want to lose'.

The breathing pattern is characterized by a decrease in the amplitude of inspiration (breath in) and an automatic stop of breathing up to 20 seconds after exhalation.

After more than 2,500 years, breathlessness continues to be a characteristic of perfection, according to the formula of Lao Tzu: 'The breath of a perfect person is as if he is not breathing at all.'

Buteyko breathing exercise 'Volitional liquidation of deep breathing' or 'The art of ephemeral, imperceptible breathing'

The descriptions of the Buteyko breathing techniques in the Glossary are presented for general reference. Please contact a specialist who is certified by the Buteyko Clinic in Moscow (est. 1987) to perform the Buteyko breathing exercises correctly. Please make sure the specialist's certificate has a logo, the signature of the copyright holder and a validity period of one year.

This is one of the simple and basic Buteyko breathing techniques (BBT) that can quickly eliminate various symptoms or aid complete recovery.

Exercise "The Art of ephemeral, imperceptible breathing"

"Volitional liquidation of deep breathing"

Try to reduce the amplitude
of breathing
REASONABLY and
SLIGHTLY.

REASONABLE - this means reducing the amplitude until you feel slight hunger for air and by only a quarter or less.

SLIGHTLY - this means that hunger for air DOES NOT CHANGE breathing pattern.

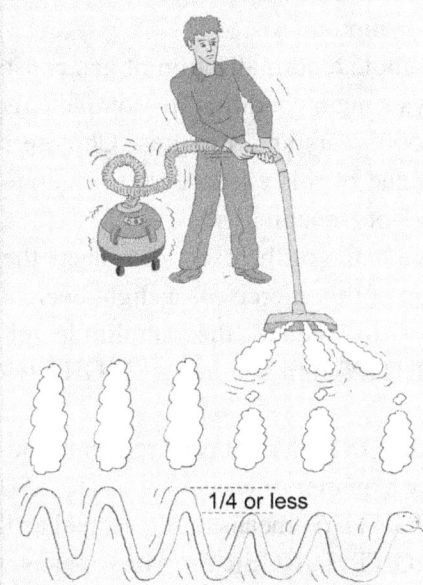

1/4 or less

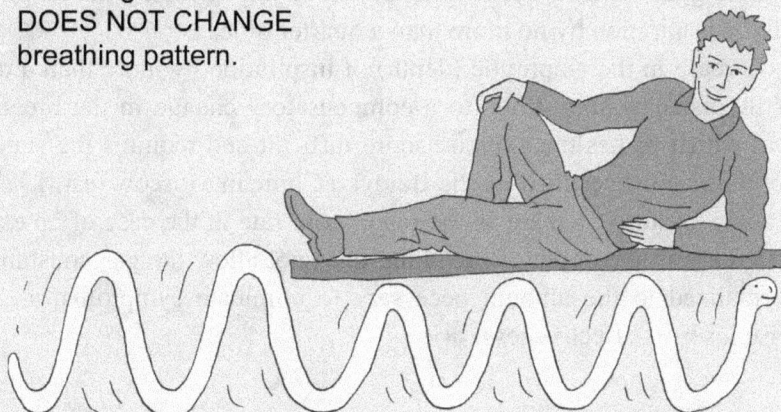

The image of a snake shows a pattern of breathing

1. Exercise 'Volitional liquidation of deep breathing' or 'The art of ephemeral, imperceptible breathing'

The elimination of the symptoms of the disease occurs gradually and depends on gas constants in the lungs and respiratory homeostasis in general.

Partial normalization of gas constants allows one to eliminate only some symptoms.

Complete normalization of gas constants and respiratory homeostasis is always a main condition for complete recovery.

2,500 years ago, the great Chinese philosopher Lao Tzu described the technique of this exercise very accurately: 'A Perfect Man Breathes As If He Is Not Breathing'.

The name of the exercise reflects the essence of the exercise. The main feature of this exercise is a slight decrease in the depth of breathing.

Try to reduce the amplitude of breathing REASONABLY and SLIGHTLY until you feel a SLIGHT HUNGER for AIR.

- REASONABLY - means reducing the amplitude or depth of breathing by only a quarter or less.
- SLIGHTLY - means until you feel a slight hunger for air.
- SLIGHT HUNGER for AIR - means without changing the breathing pattern.

The physiology of the respiratory system and the ability to adapt to changes in gas constants set a limit for effectively reducing the amplitude (depth) of inspiration by no more than a quarter or less.

A decrease in the amplitude (depth) of inspiration by more than a quarter of the usual volume leads to a compensatory change in the breathing pattern, which makes the exercise more difficult and requires the supervision of a specialist certified by the Buteyko Clinic in Moscow (est. 1987).

A compensatory increase in the respiratory rate in the case of an excessive decrease in the depth of breathing does not allow the gas constants to be normalized to the amount necessary to eliminate symptoms, and the exercise loses its effectiveness.

Exercise "Pleasant air shortage or slight hunger for air"

"Volitional liquidation of deep breathing" or the Art of ephemeral, imperceptible breathing

The image of the snake demonstrates the maintenance of the original breathing pattern during exercise.

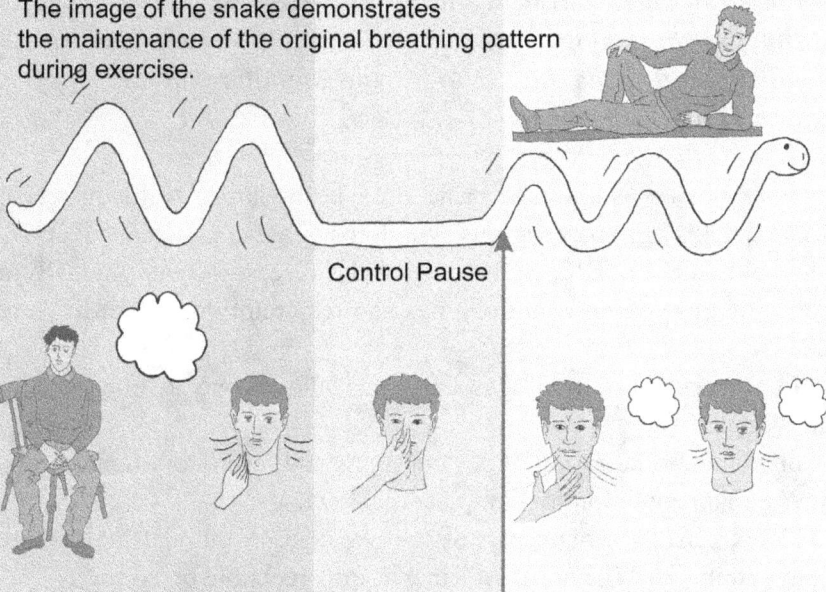

Control Pause

Short and REASONABLE breath holding, get a SLIGHT hunger for air as it happens at the end of the Control Pause.

REASONABLE - this means to get SLIGHT hunger for air.

SLIGHT hunger for air DOES NOT CHANGE original breathing pattern.

© Victor Lunn-RockLiffe (UK)
http://victorlunn-rockliffe.com/Buteyko-s-Discovery
© text by Andrey E. Novozhilov (Russia)
www.buteykomoscow.ru

2. Exercise 'Pleasant air shortage or slight hunger for air'

Buteyko breathing exercise
'A pleasant air shortage or slight hunger for air'

The descriptions of the Buteyko breathing techniques in the Glossary are presented for general reference. Please contact a specialist who is certified by the Buteyko Clinic in Moscow (est. 1987) to perform the Buteyko breathing exercises correctly. Please make sure the specialist's certificate has a logo, the signature of the copyright holder and a validity period of one year.

This is one of the simple and basic Buteyko breathing techniques (BBT) that can quickly eliminate various symptoms or aid complete recovery.

The elimination of the symptoms of the disease occurs gradually and depends on gas constants in the lungs and respiratory homeostasis in general.

Partial normalization of gas constants allows one to eliminate only some symptoms.

Complete normalization of gas constants and respiratory homeostasis is always a main condition for complete recovery.

This exercise is a main part of the exercise, 'Volitional liquidation of deep breathing' or 'The art of ephemeral, imperceptible breathing'.

Air shortage can be described as air hunger.

The goal is to find the level of pleasant air shortage which allows one to do this exercise for any length of time and without any discomfort. If the reduction of depth of each inhalation is too much, then the frequency of breathing will start increasing.

The correct performance of the exercise allows you to stop coughing and choking, and normalizes the blood pressure within a few minutes.

Correct performance means that you can reduce the amplitude (depth) of inspiration by a quarter or less.

A more significant decrease in the amplitude of inspiration will lead to a change in the initial pattern of breathing and a decrease in the effectiveness of the exercise.

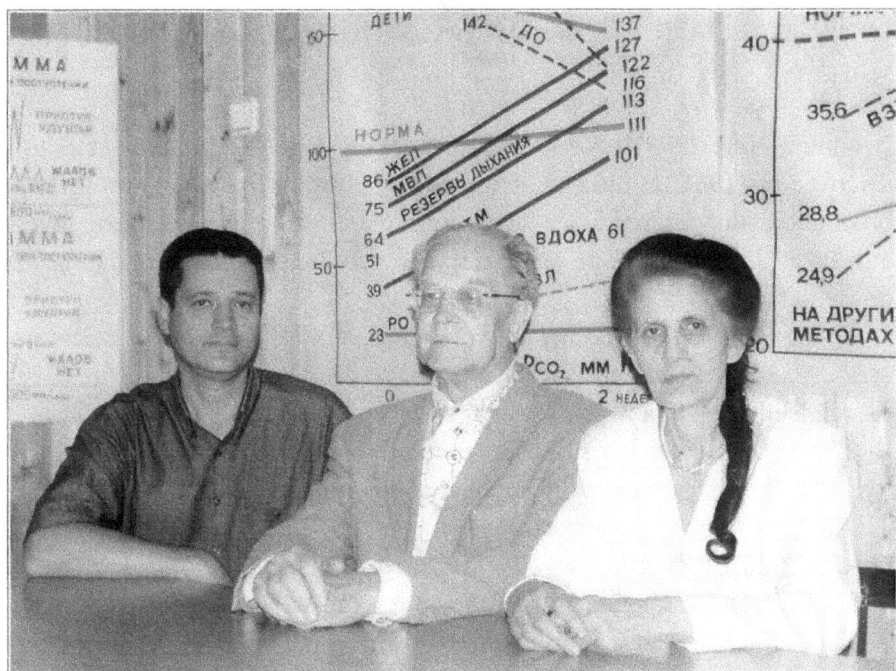

3. *Dr A. E. Novozhilov, Dr K. P. Buteyko, Dr L. D. Buteyko (Novozhilova), at the Buteyko Clinic in Moscow (est. 1987), in the 1990s*

Buteyko Clinic in Moscow (est. 1987)

It is one of the first private **medical** clinics in Moscow and Russia.

It was opened on 19 November 1987, on the basis of a decision by the government of Moscow to introduce *the Buteyko Method* into the health-care of Moscow and Russia for the treatment, prevention and recovery of various diseases.

The creators of the clinic are: Dr Konstantin Pavlovich Buteyko, author of *the Buteyko Method*, copyright holder; Dr Lyudmila Dmitrievna Buteyko (Novozhilova), co-author of *the Buteyko Method*, leading specialist, copyright holder of *the Buteyko Method* since 2003; Dr Andrey Evgenievich Novozhilov, co-author of *the Buteyko Method,* chief physician of the clinic since 1989, copyright holder since 2014.

Dr Lyudmila Dmitrievna Buteyko (Novozhilova), leading Buteyko specialist

Lyudmila Buteyko (Novozhilova) met Dr K. Buteyko and his scientific discovery in 1968, at the age of 31, when suffering from a severe form of bronchial asthma, after twice suffering clinical death as a result of severe attacks of suffocation. The emergency doctors literally spent nights in her house in those days.

Dr K. Buteyko invited her for treatment, and after having assessed her serious condition told her 9-year-old son Andrey how *to reduce breathing* to stop a choking attack and asthma, and the son cured his mother.

The choking attacks stopped completely literally in two weeks, and Lyudmila became a faithful friend and companion of Dr K. Buteyko for the next 35 years.

Lyudmila Buteyko managed to preserve the scientific discovery of Dr K. Buteyko and the personality of the author himself.

Lyudmila Buteyko was able to transform a complex medical technology into a simple and accessible form for use, known in the world as *the Buteyko Method*.

Today we know about the scientific discovery of Dr K. Buteyko and use the *Buteyko Method* thanks exclusively to Lyudmila Buteyko.

A legend claims that Lyudmila Buteyko could stop a cough or an attack of suffocation in a patient with bronchial asthma simply by talking to them on the phone, and her art of *reducing breathing* or teaching children to breathe according to Buteyko used to produce amazement.

Andrey Evgenievich Novozhilov, MD, chief physician of the Buteyko Clinic in Moscow

Dr A. Novozhilov was born and grew up in Moscow. He is a graduate of the Sechenov First Moscow State Medical University with a degree in *Medical Science, General Medicine*.

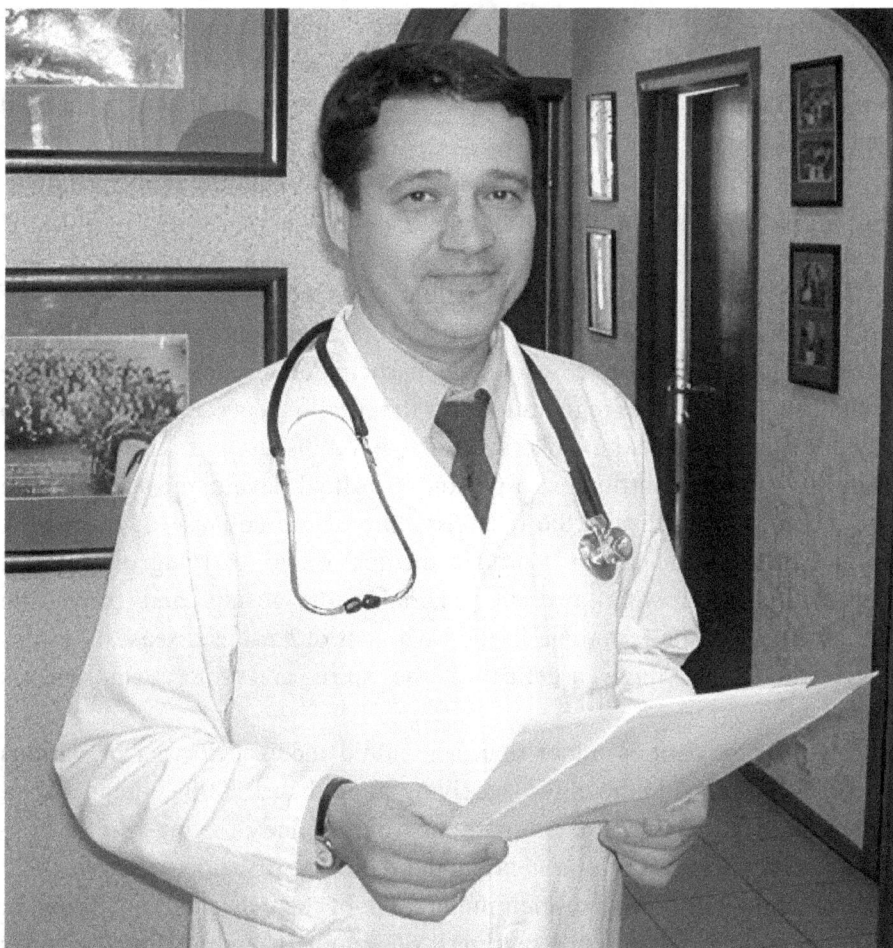

4. Dr Andrey E. Novozhilov, chief physician of the Buteyko Clinic in Moscow (est. 1987), co-author of the Buteyko Method, copyright holder, 2005

Since 1989, he has been the chief physician of the Buteyko Clinic. He is the author of a unique programme for the treatment of bronchial asthma with the help of physical exercises under the control of breathing. It allows former asthmatics to return to active life and cure any form of the disease, regardless of its severity and prescription.

The reference book *Who's Who* includes information about the chief physician of the Buteyko Clinic in Moscow, Dr A. Novozhilov: the head of a commercial medical institution who has been working for more than 20 years in Russia.

For all those years, the clinic has been operating on the basis of a medical licence specializing on therapy and paediatrics, issued by the Moscow Department of Health.

In the history of the Buteyko Clinic in Moscow, there are names of people whose work has brought fame and state recognition to the Buteyko Method, names of people who have participated in state testing of the technique and in the registration of the first patents for the Buteyko Method. There are also members who have led discussions on whether the Buteyko Method contributes to personal spiritual development. And there are members who during the troubled time of the collapse of the USSR were effectively managing a private medical clinic, carrying out clinical observations and were able to generalize the results and prove the effectiveness of the technique in the treatment of various diseases; besides much more that these ascetics of the spirit and sincere enthusiasts achieved.

In different periods, more than a hundred medical doctors of various specialties worked in the clinic, receiving more than 10,000 patients a year, which allowed them to accumulate vast experience in using *the Buteyko Method* for the treatment, prevention and recovery of various diseases.

The clinic has a unique scientific archive of the author, Dr K. Buteyko: a large archive of video recordings of seminars and practical classes conducted by Dr K. Buteyko and a leading specialist, Dr L. Buteyko (Novozhilova). It makes the clinic a recognized leader in training new specialists in the application of *the Buteyko Method* in Russia and around the world.

Confirmation of the relevant training and qualifications of teachers of *the Buteyko Method* is a Specialist Certificate, which necessarily contains the logo of the Buteyko Clinic in Moscow, the signature of the copyright holder and has a validity period of one year.

The certificate is renewed annually, which guarantees the high qualification of the teacher of *the Buteyko Method*.

The official website of the Buteyko Clinic in Moscow (est. 1987) is www.buteykomoscow.ru

Buteyko Konstantin Pavlovich (1923–2003)

Russian doctor, scientist, philosopher, author of the theory of degradation and death of modern civilization as a result of the spread of the 'deep breathing' disease.

He is **author of the scientific discovery** of the *'deep breathing' disease* and the creator of a drug-free method of treatment known as *the Buteyko Method*.

He is **author of the theory of degradation and death of modern civilization** as a result of the spread of the *'deep breathing' disease*.

Deep breathing disease as a cause of degradation and death of modern civilization

Dr K. Buteyko has scientifically proven the existence of the *deep breathing disease*, deciphered its mechanism and invented a drug-free method of treatment known as *the Buteyko Method*.

Dr K. Buteyko has argued that the *deep breathing disease* is the cause of the rapid spread of the so-called diseases of civilization (asthma, allergies, hypertension, atherosclerosis, diabetes, mental and nervous diseases, oncology and others), which today account for 90% of cases of general morbidity.

Dr K. Buteyko has clinically proven that the use of *the Buteyko Method* in therapeutic, preventive and wellness practices not only cures the so-called diseases of civilization, but also prevents their occurrence in risk groups.

For example, *the Buteyko Method* can cure bronchial asthma practically without drugs, with the help of breathing techniques and physical exercises under the control of breathing. The state clinical approbation of *the Buteyko Method* (Sechenov First Moscow State Medical University, 1983,

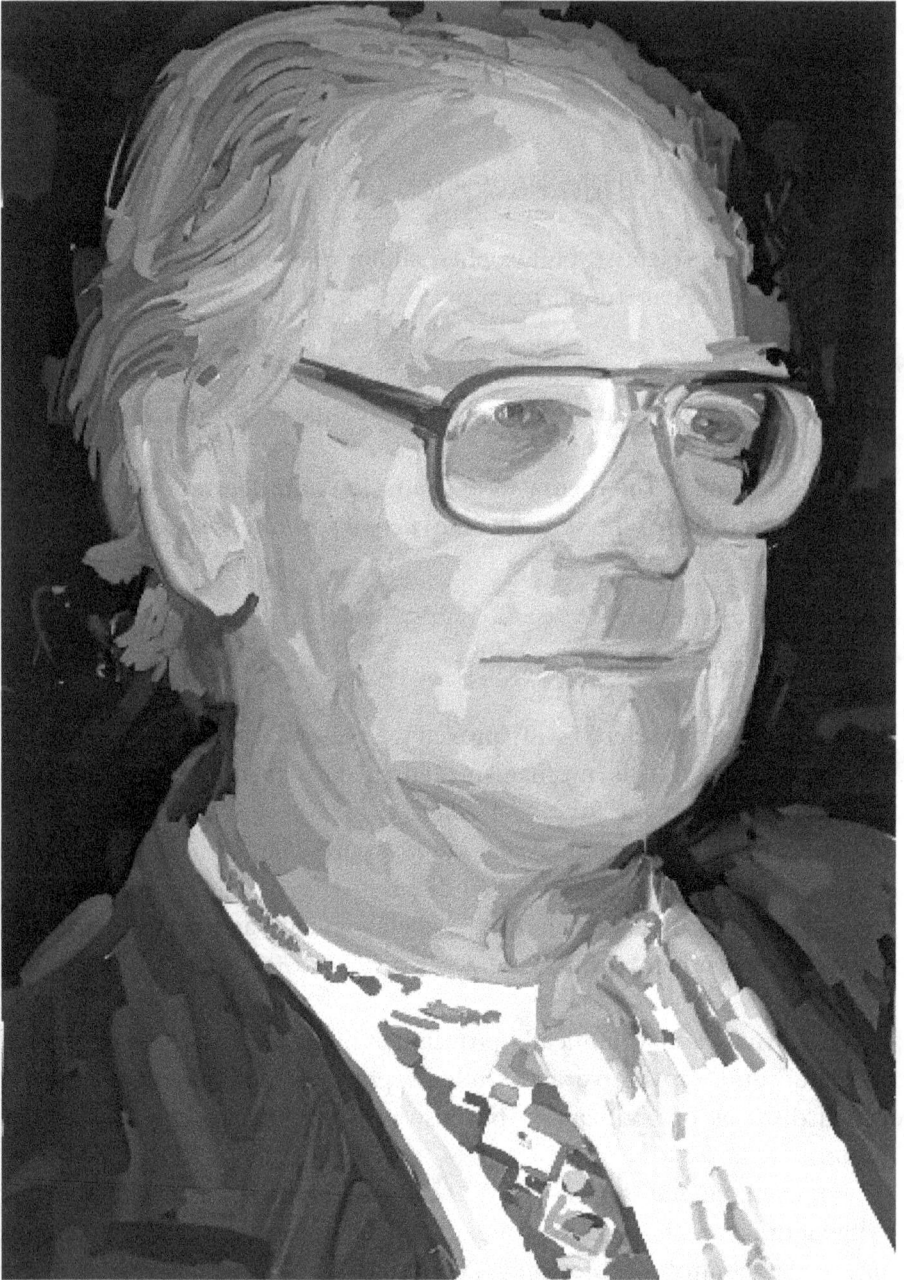

5. *Dr Konstantin P. Buteyko, 2000, New Zealand, ©Victor Lunn-Rockliffe*
http://victorlunn-rockliffe.com/Buteyko-s-Discovery

Russia) showed that children practising Buteyko breathing not only got rid of bronchial asthma, but also **stopped getting sick with viral diseases and colds.**

Dr K. Buteyko argued that the *deep breathing disease* is the cause of the degradation of personality, degradation and death of modern civilization.

Dr K. Buteyko argued that the *deep breathing disease*, creating chronic hypoxia of the cerebral cortex responsible for intelligent activity, is the cause of the degradation of a reasonable personality, which is expressed in the predominance of subcortical instincts characteristic of animal behavior (sexual, food, aggression).

The predominance of subcortical instincts turns reasonable human activity directed at the study and development of the surrounding world into aggressive and destructive forms, which will inevitably lead to the death of civilization as a result of poisoning and destruction of the habitat (industrial chemistry, herbicides, antibiotics, wars, etc.).

Dr K. Buteyko pointed out that modern civilization has a planetary character, therefore the death of civilization threatens the existence of humanity as a biological species.

He was born on 27 January 1923, in the village of Ivannitsa, near Kiev, Ukraine (USSR).

He lived and worked in Russia in the Research Institute of Experimental Biology and Medicine of the USSR Academy of Sciences (Novosibirsk, Akademgorodok), in the private medical clinic 'Breathing by Buteyko' (Novosibirsk, Akademgorodok) and in the private medical 'Buteyko Clinic' in Moscow.

After the collapse of the USSR in 1991, he became a citizen of Ukraine.

He died on 2 May 2003 in Moscow, and was buried in the Crimea, in Feodosia, the village of Beregovoe.

Dr K. Buteyko was a participant and veteran of the Second World War, having spent four years at the front. Every year, on 9 May, the Victory Day for World War II, Dr K. Buteyko, as a veteran, received personal congratulations from the President of Ukraine.

After the end of World War II, he graduated with honours from the Sechenov First Moscow State Medical University. He was the best student

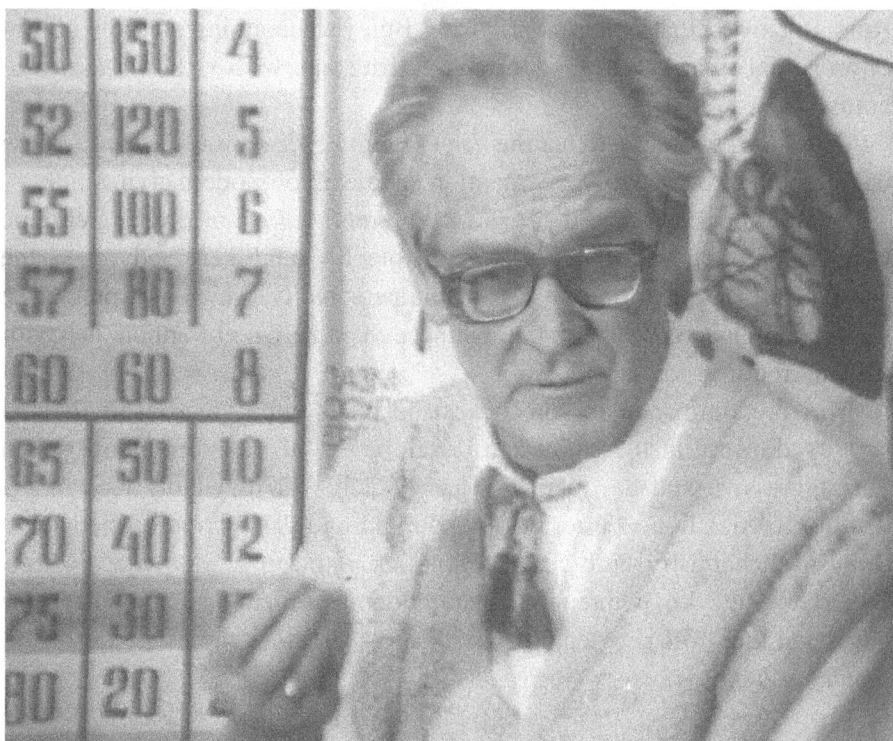

6. Dr Konstantin P. Buteyko in a frame from the film "Dr Buteyko's friends and enemies", Sverdlovsk Film Studio, 1988

of Academician Evgeny M. Tareev, on whose recommendation, as a leading specialist, he was sent to work for Academician Evgeny N. Meshalkin at the Institute of Experimental Biology and Medicine of the USSR Academy of Sciences in Novosibirsk. There for 10 years he led the scientific laboratory he created with unique equipment, where he scientifically substantiated his discovery of *deep breathing disease* and the method of its treatment, known as *the Buteyko Method*.

He was author of more than a hundred scientific publications, several scientific discoveries and inventions, including the adaptation of the human organism to tenfold flight overload and prolonged stay at great depth.

After a report by the Scientific Council of the USSR Ministry of Health, the scientific topic of *deep breathing disease* was closed, as being contrary to the scientific trends and ambitions of medical officials of those years, and Buteyko's laboratory was physically destroyed. According to stories from friends and colleagues, Dr K. Buteyko turned grey that evening; he became grey not in the war, not on the firing line, but after the destruction of his scientific laboratory.

Dr K. Buteyko continued to fight for his scientific discovery, giving public and scientific lectures. As a result, since the early 1970s, Dr K. Buteyko was included on the so-called 'black list' of scientists. These were public and political figures whose scientific works were banned from publication in the USSR, and previously published works were withdrawn from libraries and destroyed because of their pronounced opposition to the scientific ambitions of medical officials and their divergence from the socio-political trends in society of those years.

According to Dr K. Buteyko himself, the nationwide recognition and gratitude of the patients he cured, among whom were many high-ranking individuals from law enforcement agencies, helped him to keep going during that difficult period of scientific silence, the lies around his name and the scientific persecution.

Also the incredible love and support of his loyal friend and colleague, Lyudmila Dmitrievna Buteyko (Novozhilova) with whom he lived together for the rest of his life, almost 40 years, helped him to survive. Lyudmila Buteyko managed not only to save the scientific discoveries of Dr K. Buteyko and the personality of the author himself, but Lyudmila Buteyko was able to transform a complex scientific technology, incomprehensible to many medical doctors, into a simple and accessible form for use, known in the world as *the Buteyko Method*.

The fact that today we know about the scientific discovery of Dr K. Buteyko, which saved, without exaggeration, millions of human lives, and the fact that today we can use the Buteyko Method, is solely thanks to Lyudmila Buteyko.

In those years, Dr K. Buteyko was greatly supported by the mass media. The central press of those years periodically published publications 'about the legendary, mysterious scientist from Siberia, who invented a drug-free method of treating all diseases'.

There were many legends about *the Buteyko Method* in the country, Dr K. Buteyko himself receiving up to 200 letters a day asking for help. He never charged a fee for medical admission or treatment; patients paid as much as they could and were grateful for it.

Changes in the last years of the USSR allowed them to open the Buteyko Clinic in Moscow in 1987, the creators of which are Dr K. Buteyko himself, Dr L. Buteyko (Novozhilova) and Dr A. Novozhilov, chief physician there from the day it opened.

The Buteyko Clinic in Moscow received up to 10,000 patients a year. More than 100 medical doctors of various specialties worked there, which allowed us to accumulate vast experience in using *the Buteyko Method* in the treatment of various diseases and in creating unique training programmes for new specialists.

Dr K. Buteyko, Dr L. Buteyko (Novozhilova) and Dr A. Novozhilov were participants at the First International Conference dedicated to *the Buteyko Method* in New Zealand in 2000.

Additional information is available on the website of the Buteyko Clinic in Moscow: https://www.buteykomoscow.ru/bkp/

Buteyko Method

A *medical technology* of drug-free prevention and treatment of diseases resulting from violations of *respiratory homeostasis* and the action of *homeostatic (stabilizing) reactions of the functional respiratory system*, as well as other organism systems of various levels, from metabolic to behavioural, whose normal operation is functionally related to the respiratory system.

Three components of the Buteyko Method

1. Legendary breathing techniques, the qualified use of which normalizes *gas constants* and *respiratory homeostasis* only as a result of the normalization of pulmonary ventilation or so-called *external respiration*.

2. The use of dosed physical activity under the control of breathing, which allows the use of muscle activity as a natural mechanism for the normalization of *gas constants and respiratory homeostasis*.
3. The formation of a fine, artful and high level of sensitivity to breathing, which allows you to understand and feel changes in *external respiration* (pulmonary ventilation) under the influence of various factors and to prevent the occurrence of various symptoms or diseases.

The Buteyko Method as a method of treatment cannot be reduced to just holding your breath or to any breathing exercises, as some ignorant people suppose.

The fact is that *respiratory homeostasis* (the constancy of respiratory gases) is supported by both ventilation of the lungs (the so-called *external respiration*) and normal activity of the general metabolism.

In order to normalize *gas constants and respiratory homeostasis*, we can arbitrarily change the ventilation of the lungs (breathing techniques) and influence the activity of metabolism with the help of dosed muscle work (walking, elementary sports).

Muscle work is a natural mechanism for regulating *respiratory homeostasis*, and if this natural mechanism is not used, then possible changes in *external respiration* (pulmonary ventilation) under the influence of various factors will need to be constantly compensated through the help of breathing techniques.

The formation of a fine, artful and high level of sensitivity to changes in pulmonary ventilation is of significant help in various situations, which makes it possible to prevent violations of *respiratory homeostasis* effectively with the help of either muscle activity (walking, elementary sports), or with the help of simple breathing techniques.

Medical technology

From the ancient Greek *technos* and *logos*, meaning art, skill, knowledge. It is a series of sequential actions aimed at introducing scientific knowledge into medical practice.

Physiological functional respiratory system

A self-organizing and self-regulating complex of individual components in order to maintain the optimal level of oxygen (pO_2), carbon dioxide (pCO_2) and acid-based equilibrium (pH) for metabolism.

1. The fundamental scientific research of Dr K. Buteyko was the development of the scientific theory of the Russian physiologist, academician, Professor Peter K. Anokhin, according to which the human organism is a complex of self-organizing and self-regulating physiological functional systems, the normal operation of which ensures the maintenance of constant physiological values. It allows the organism, as a so-called *open system*, to maintain the constancy of the internal environment - *homeostasis*.

The mechanism of self-regulation of the functional system of the organism forms *stabilizing (homeostatic) reactions* that occur when *constants* are changed, and get eliminated by themselves as homeostasis normalizes.

The normal operation of the entire complex of functional systems of the organism ensures *health*.

The physiology of *the functional systems of the organism* unites individual organs into systems not according to anatomical features and location, as is customary in classical physiology, but according to the tasks for which such an association of systems and organs is intended.

For example, in order to maintain the vital constants of oxygen (O_2) and carbon dioxide (CO_2) in the cells of the organism, a physiological *functional respiratory system* has been formed, which consists of an *external respiratory* system (the ventilation of the pulmonary alveoli) and a circulatory system that ensures the transfer of respiratory gases from the lungs to the cells.

In this case, anatomically different formations - the respiratory organs and the circulatory system - are combined into a functional system to perform a common task: maintaining gas *constants* (CO_2 and O_2) and *respiratory homeostasis* in the lungs, the blood and the cells.

«In the process of evolution, environmental conditions were changed and *functional physiological systems* were formed that ensured the maintenance of *constants* within the normal range. For example, a complex functional respiratory system has been formed to maintain such vital *constants* as oxygen (O_2) and carbon dioxide (CO_2) in the cell.

At first, respiration was carried out by simple diffusion of gases through the shell of a single-celled organism. With the formation of multicellular organisms, it became necessary to transfer gases from the surface layers of the organism to the internal areas. In particular, for this purpose, the blood and circulatory system was formed as a transport site of the functional respiratory system. And only later, as the structures and functions of the organism became more complicated, a functional system of external respiration was formed which provides ventilation of the alveoli of the lungs in contact with blood.

The ultimate goal of the entire respiratory system is to maintain O_2 and CO_2 in cells and tissues at a normal level.

Respiratory homeostasis is the constancy of the gas composition of blood and tissues.» (Dr K. Buteyko, 'Regulation of bronchial tone (tonus) in healthy and patients with bronchial asthma'. Institute of Physiology of the Siberian Branch of the USSR Academy of Sciences, Novosibirsk, Akademgorodok, 1967, manuscript)

2. Violation of *respiratory homeostasis* as a result of changes in vital gas *constants* forms *homeostatic (stabilizing) reactions of the physiological functional respiratory system*, which act until the normalization of *constants* and are able to eliminate themselves as *homeostasis* gets normalized.

3. Scientific research by Dr K. Buteyko has shown that the effect of homeostatic reactions forms a clinical picture of diseases of organs and systems, often anatomically unrelated, but which take part in the construction of the functional system of the organism. Its work is disrupted and does not maintain *constants* and *homeostasis*.

4. Scientific research by Dr K. Buteyko has established an inverse relationship between a decrease in CO_2 in the lungs and an increase in uneven ventilation of the lungs, which leads to the appearance of symptoms of *bronchospasm* in diseases occurring with increased bronchial tone, while normalization of the CO_2 *constant* in the lungs leads to the elimination of *bronchospasm*.

A decrease in CO_2 in the lungs is the cause of *metabolic hypoxia*, oxygen deficiency in cells, in metabolism, which can be the cause of vascular spasm, the cause of *peripheral angiospasm* and an increase in blood pressure.

Bronchospasm and arterial hypertension can be eliminated by themselves as the CO_2 *constant* in the lungs normalizes. It allows us to consider them as physiological *homeostatic reactions of the functional respiratory system*, the action of which is aimed at normalizing *respiratory homeostasis*.

5. Dr K. Buteyko identified two reasons for the reduction of CO_2 in the lungs and the appearance of symptoms of *bronchospasm* or hypertension:
• *chronic hyperventilation of the lungs (deep breathing)*;
• *hypodynamia* or prolonged inactivity.

6. A graphic recording of breathing in patients with *chronic hyperventilation of the lungs* shows an increase in the depth of breathing with a slight change in other parameters, on the basis of which Dr K. Buteyko introduced the term 'deep breathing' and announced *the therapeutic principle of the Buteyko Method - a gradual decrease of the depth of breathing to normal*.

7. *The Buteyko Method* as a method of prevention and treatment is based on the normalization of *respiratory homeostasis* with the help of special breathing techniques, with the help of muscular (physical) exercises under the control of breathing and the formation of fine sensitivity to changes in lung ventilation in any situation.

The therapeutic principle of the Buteyko Method

This principle is the gradual decrease of the depth of breathing to normal. 'Principle' comes from the Latin *principium*, meaning the first, the basis, the beginning, on the basis of which subsequent actions are created.

The graphic recording of breathing in patients with *chronic hyperventilation of the lungs* shows an increase in the depth of breathing with a slight change in other parameters, on the basis of which Dr K. Buteyko suggests normalizing the depth (amplitude) of breathing.

The arbitrary change in other breathing parameters (frequency, duration of inhalation or exhalation, etc.) with the help of special breathing techniques does not allow one to normalize *gas constants, respiratory homeostasis* and prevent the occurrence of *homeostatic reactions of the functional respiratory system*.

The breathing techniques of the Buteyko Method, created on the basis of this principle, in the process of their implementation make it possible to eliminate the symptoms of *bronchospasm*, stop coughing, normalize blood pressure, which leads to significant clinical improvement and recovery as *gas constants and respiratory homeostasis* get normalized.

The therapeutic principle of the Buteyko Method - a gradual decrease of the depth of breathing to normal - was not previously known, nor described nor found in the available literature. It is the invention of Dr K. Buteyko and is the basis of the drug-free method of treatment known as the Buteyko Method.

The range of application of the Buteyko Method

The spectrum of application of the Buteyko Method covers more than **150 diseases of the respiratory system, blood circulation, metabolism and immunity**, which today account for 90% of cases of morbidity and belong to the so-called 'diseases of civilization', including **bronchial asthma, bronchitis, allergies, rhinitis and sinusitis, high blood pressure, angina, diabetes** and others.

The Buteyko Method makes it possible to effectively treat and prevent the occurrence of diseases of organs and systems, the normal operation of which is functionally related to breathing, and these are **chronic fatigue, stress, sleep disorders, snoring, sleep apnea, post-Covid syndrome** and others.

Qualified application of the Buteyko Method by a specialist with a certificate from the Buteyko Clinic in Moscow (est. 1987) allows one to eliminate the acute symptoms of disease during the lesson and increase the *control or maximum pause* by 5 or more seconds, which indicates effective treatment.

The formula of the Buteyko Method, created by Dr Buteyko himself

Dr Buteyko said that his method is like a magic pill in your head, which is always with you and which will always help. Therefore, Dr Buteyko outlined the essence of his method in the so-called 'rule of the left hand': the hand that is closer to the heart.

THE ESSENCE OF BUTEYKO

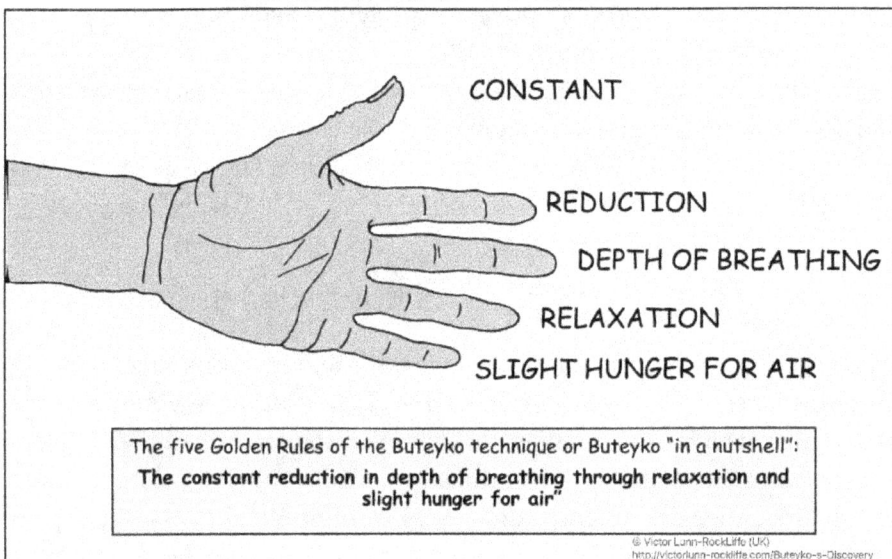

CONSTANT

REDUCTION

DEPTH OF BREATHING

RELAXATION

SLIGHT HUNGER FOR AIR

The five Golden Rules of the Buteyko technique or Buteyko "in a nutshell":
The constant reduction in depth of breathing through relaxation and slight hunger for air"

© Victor Lunn-RockLiffe (UK)
http://victorlunn-rockliffe.com/Buteyko-s-Discovery

7. The essence of the Buteyko Method is the so-called 'rule of the left hand', the hand that is closer to the heart.

In this rule, each word corresponds to one finger of the hand and explains what needs to be done for recovery:

• reducing (thumb, or this word means what to do);

• the depth (index finger of the hand, or this word explains that only the depth can be changed in the breath);

• of breathing (middle finger of the hand);

- relaxation (ring finger of the hand, or this word explains how to reduce the depth of breathing);

- to a slight hunger for air (little finger of the hand, or these words explain how you can understand that you have really reduced the depth of breathing).

Dr Buteyko always added that air hunger should be small, like this smallest finger of the hand. A slight hunger for air means without changing the pattern of breathing.

The Buteyko Method is about relaxation and a constant reduction of breathing

In practice, the success of treatment largely depends on the individual sensitivity of the patient to their own breathing. So the co-author of the technique, Dr L. Buteyko (Novozhilova), proposed the following definition: "The Buteyko Method is a sort of fine (artful, sophisticated, high) sensitivity to changes in the depth of breathing. It is the ability to understand, feel and know one's own breathing in order to consciously change and normalize it. The main mechanisms in the Buteyko Method are the natural mechanisms of normalization of breathing - relaxation, correct posture and **automatic** reduction of the depth of breathing."

There are no breathing exercises in the Buteyko Method

Dr K. Buteyko suggested using natural mechanisms of normalization of the depth of breathing, which consist in correct posture, in muscle relaxation, the tone of which affects breathing, in muscular (physical) exercises under the breathing control.

Once I heard about a man aged 90 living in New York who had a *control pause* of 90 seconds. He said, «The secret of my health is simple. In the 1970s I listened to a lecture by Dr K. Buteyko himself and remembered that *deep breathing* is the cause of diseases, and that relaxation reduces and normalizes breathing. I realized that there are no breathing exercises in the Buteyko Method, but only relaxation and reduction of breathing:

an automatic reduction of breathing, which occurs by itself as a result of relaxation. Each time I remembered Buteyko, each time I relaxed. The main thing is to feel how the breathing decreases.»

The Law of Death is deep breathing

Dr K. Buteyko said, "I managed to discover and mathematically describe The Law of Death: the deeper the breath, the closer the death of the organism. To make a person sick, it is enough to teach him to constantly breathe deeply; this is scarier than any weapon.

Deep breathing will destroy the metabolism, then the immune system, and the organism will die. But first the protective mechanisms from *deep breathing* will start to work: the nose will stop breathing, bronchial spasm will appear, suffocation, blood pressure will increase.

If the effectiveness of these protective mechanisms turns out to be low or we eliminate them with the help of drugs, then the lungs will collapse, pneumofibrosis will appear, and the vessels will be filled with cholesterol plaque."

The Law of Life is breathlessness

"I managed to decipher the ancient Law of Life, announced in the tradition of yoga: *breathlessness* is immortality."

The formula of health

"I managed to explain the physiological essence of the Formula of Health, voiced by the brilliant Lao Tzu 2,500 years ago: 'The breath of a perfect person is as if he is not breathing at all.'

Our task is not only to discover and decipher the secrets of *health* and longevity, to create a mathematical description of the Disease Formula and the Health Formula, but to make this knowledge available to people and put this knowledge at the service of people."

(Dr K. Buteyko, transcript of the video recording of the seminar for specialists, Buteyko Clinic in Moscow, 1990, manuscript)

Control Pause (CP)

This is the voluntary *apnea* after exhalation, which is performed without volitional effort, an indicator of which is the normal amplitude (depth) of the first breath after the end of *apnea*, as well as the preservation of the original breathing pattern without significant changes.

It is measured in seconds and requires high sensitivity to breathing.

It is used to measure the CO_2 *constant* in the lungs according to the table of Dr K. Buteyko.

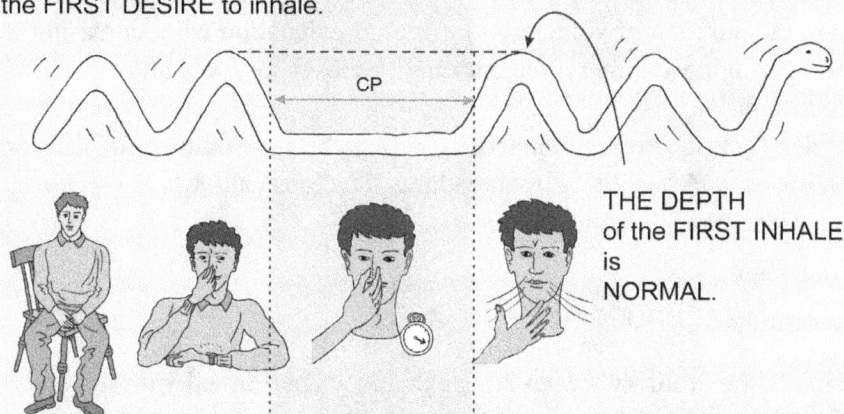

How to measure Control Pause (CP)

After a NORMAL exhalation, stop breathing and do not breathe until
the FIRST DESIRE to inhale.

CP

THE DEPTH
of the FIRST INHALE
is
NORMAL.

The duration of voluntary breath holding (CP) should be REASONABLE.

REASONABLE - this means that the depth of breathing has not increased and pattern of the breathing has not changed after measuring CP.

Normal CP is 45 seconds, which indicates normal CO2 pressure in the lungs and the absence of excessive breathing and deep breathing disease.

8. How to measure CP

With *deep breathing*, the CO_2 pressure in the lungs decreases, which is the cause of *metabolic hypoxia*, which, in turn, is the cause of a decrease in the duration of voluntary *apnea* after exhalation.

A CP of 45 seconds corresponds to the normal pressure of CO_2 in the alveoli of the lungs, equal to 40 mm Hg. However, Dr K. Buteyko considered this indicator underestimated due to the presence of some symptoms of diseases.

Dr K. Buteyko pointed out that the 'bearing constant' of the CO_2 *constant* in the lungs, in which there are no symptoms of known diseases, shows 60 seconds on CP as the lower limit of the norm.

He noted that without a certain experience, everyone measures the duration of *apnea* with some volitional effort, which is characteristic of measuring the *maximum pause (MP)*, and suggests that *apnea* measured in this way be called *the maximum pause* for novice practitioners of *the Buteyko Method* and *the control pause* for experienced practitioners.

The development of sensitivity to breathing makes it possible to measure the duration of voluntary *apnea* after exhalation with increasing accuracy, bringing the measurement quality closer to the characteristic of the control pause.

Dr K. Buteyko recommended starting the measurement of the control pause as the sensitivity to breathing develops and when *the maximum pause* increases to 25 to 30 seconds.

Maximum Pause (MP)

This is the arbitrary *apnea* after exhalation, performed with a slight volitional effort, an indicator of which is a slight increase in the frequency and depth of breathing after the end of the measurement.

At the initial stage of treatment, it can be used instead of a *control pause* as a way to assess the dynamics of CO_2 in the lungs and the effectiveness of classes.

Dr K. Buteyko pointed out that the lesson is considered effective if the symptoms of the disease are eliminated, and in their absence if the *control* or *maximum* pause is increased by five or more seconds.

Control Pause (CP) &
Maximum Pause (MP)

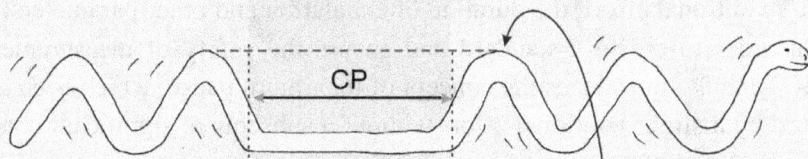

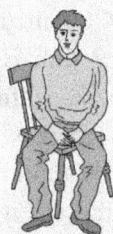

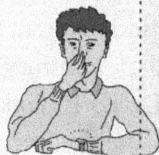

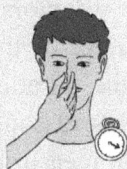

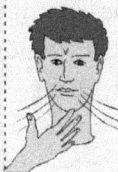

CP

NORMAL depth
of the FIRST BREATH
after
CP measurement

The main feature of the Control Pause (CP)
is the presence
of the normal depth of breathing after measurement.

If the depth of the first inhalation is increased,
then this is called
the Maximum Pause (MP).

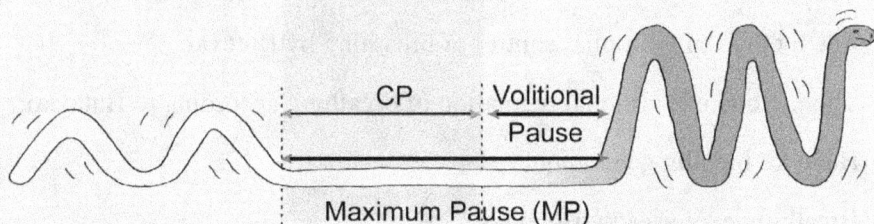

CP

Volitional
Pause

Maximum Pause (MP)

9. Control and Maximum Pauses

In some manuscripts, Dr K. Buteyko talks about measuring the maximum breath retention (breath hold) after exhalation, *apnea* after exhalation, without providing an accurate description of the measurement method, since the duration of *apnea* can vary significantly depending on the patient's volitional effort, the duration of exhalation and other parameters.

In order to create a standard and ensure the safety of measurements, Dr K. Buteyko introduces the concept of maximum pause, which is characterized by a slight volitional effort without a subsequent significant change in the breathing pattern.

The sensitivity of the respiratory receptors to changes in CO_2 in the lungs allows you to notice the dynamics of the indicator in 1.2 mm Hg, which corresponds to a change in the duration of arbitrary *apnea* after exhalation by about 5 seconds. For this reason, Dr K. Buteyko repeatedly pointed out that excessive accuracy in measuring the control or maximum pause is not required, since a therapeutic and diagnostic value has the dynamics of the indicator by 5 seconds.

Other names of the Buteyko Method that reflect only one part of it are breathing techniques

The Buteyko Method has common synonyms of the name:

- The method of VLGD (volitional elimination of deep breathing),

- The method of volitional control of breathing by Buteyko,

- The method of volitional regulation of breathing according to Buteyko,

- Buteyko breathing techniques,

- Breathing exercises by Buteyko,

- Breathing exercises of the Buteyko Method,

- Breathing by Buteyko.

Two conditions for a successful specialist of the Buteyko Method

Dr K. Buteyko said that in order to become a qualified teacher of the Buteyko Method, it is necessary to fulfil two conditions:

First of all, cure any disease in yourself. Doctor, heal yourself!

Secondly, if you are healthy and did not have the opportunity to learn from your own experience how *to reduce breathing*, then as soon as your patient stops coughing, stops a choking attack, or eliminates nasal congestion, then from that moment you, having discarded pride and warning, should learn from your talented patient the art of *reducing breathing*.

Dr K. Buteyko said that many people, but not all, have a natural sensitivity to breathing and are able to reduce the depth of breathing, despite your explanations and even contrary to your explanations of how it should be done.

Learn from such reasonable patients how to reduce breathing correctly, and you will also stop getting sick.

If the patient is not able *to reduce breathing*, and you will soon see this, then teach them to perform volitional breath hold properly, and the disease will go away.

It happens that the patient cannot or does not want to eliminate the causes of *deep breathing*, and does not want or does not know how *to reduce breathing*. In this case, strong-willed breath holds will help in the treatment, although they do not allow one to get rid of the disease completely.

Strong-willed breath holds eliminate the symptoms of the disease, but do not develop a fine sensitivity to breathing, do not allow us to feel how our breathing changes under the influence of various events and factors, and therefore do not allow us to find the causes of our *deep breathing*.

Dr K. Buteyko often repeated that the organism is a 'black box'. There is such a thing in physics: a black box with an input signal and an output signal, and no one knows what happens inside the box and how the output signal is formed.

Today we know that CO_2 in the lungs regulates muscle tone in the bronchial wall and affects the activity of *allergic inflammation of the bronchi*. This knowledge makes it possible to treat bronchial asthma successfully using a sophisticated medical technology called *the Buteyko Method*.

But we do not know how these processes are carried out; this is a task for future scientific research.

Copyright in the Buteyko Method

The Buteyko Method was created on the basis of a scientific discovery and invention in medicine made by Dr Konstantin P. Buteyko on 7 October 1952 in Moscow.

The co-authors are Dr Lyudmila D. Buteyko (Russia, Moscow) and Dr Andrey E. Novozhilov (Russia, Moscow).

The Buteyko Method is an intellectual property and an object of copyright (patents №№ 1067640, 1593627, 224517, registered trademarks БУТЕЙКО (Rus), BUTEYKO (Eng) №№ 367700, 379371, 103540, WIPO 1009432).

State clinical studies have demonstrated a significant impact of the Buteyko Method on the human organism and health; therefore, according to the decision of the author, co-authors and copyright holders, the use of the Buteyko Method or any part of it is possible only after special training.

Please contact a specialist who is certified by the Buteyko Clinic in Moscow (est. 1987) to perform the Buteyko breathing exercises correctly.

The Specialist's Certificate is a confirmation of qualification and permission to use the Buteyko Method.

The Specialist's Certificate has a logo, the signature of the copyright holder and a validity period of one year.

The copyright in the Buteyko Method has one goal, which is quality: high-quality teacher training and high-quality advisory support for teachers.

Bronchial obstruction reversible

This is the reversible reduction in the diameter of the bronchi due to oedema, hypersecretion of sputum and *bronchospasm*.

The clinical manifestation of bronchial obstruction depends on the predominance of any of its components, for example, oedema is wheezing, excessive sputum is wheezing, *bronchospasm* is suffocation.

Chronic allergic inflammation of the bronchi and asthma

According to the generally accepted theory, bronchial asthma occurs due to chronic allergic inflammation of the bronchi, the activity of which forms the clinical picture of reversible bronchial obstruction and all bronchial asthma.

According to *the CO_2-deficient theory of bronchial asthma* proposed by Dr K. Buteyko, allergic inflammation of the bronchi is **a part of the mechanism** of reversible bronchial obstruction, **but is not its cause**.

Allergic inflammation of the bronchi occurs when the CO_2 *constant* in the lungs changes and increases simultaneously with an increase in *alveolar hypocapnia*, which is accompanied by an increase in clinical manifestations of bronchial obstruction and asthma.

It is completely eliminated when the CO_2 *constant* in the lungs is normalized.

Bronchospasm (bronchial spasm)

This is a reversible decrease in the diameter of the bronchi as a result of an increase in the tone of the smooth muscles of the bronchial wall.

It is a component of reversible bronchial obstruction; it occurs with a decrease in CO_2 in the lungs; it acts until partial or complete normalization of this *constant*; and is able to be eliminated automatically as *respiratory homeostasis* normalizes.

This forms the clinical picture of *deep breathing disease*. Drug elimination of reversible bronchial obstruction without normalization of *gas constants* is the cause of the rapid development of pneumofibrosis, which is an irreversible *homeostatic reaction of the functional respiratory system*.

Discovered by the Russian scientist Dr K. Buteyko in the mid-1970s, the inverse relationship between CO_2 in the lungs and increased bronchial tone in diseases occurring with increased bronchial tone made it possible to create **a fundamentally new theory of bronchial asthma**, according to which a deficiency of CO_2 in the lungs *(alveolar hypocapnia)* is the cause of chronic allergic inflammation of the bronchi, bronchospasm and bronchial obstruction.

For the occurrence of bronchial obstruction in patients with asthma, chronic allergic inflammation of the bronchi is formed, the cause of which is *alveolar hypocapnia*.

The long-term clinical application of *the Buteyko Method* for the treatment of diseases occurring with reversible bronchial obstruction (asthma, bronchitis, etc.) has convincingly shown that the elimination of *alveolar hypocapnia* and normalization of the CO_2 *constant* in the lungs makes it impossible to provoke bronchospasm and other manifestations of bronchial obstruction, on the basis of which we can talk about the elimination of chronic allergic inflammation of the bronchi.

Today we can observe numerous cases of remission of bronchial asthma lasting 30 to 50 years.

The complete absence of any manifestations of bronchial asthma with the normalization of the CO_2 *constant* in the lungs allows us to consider bronchospasm as a *stabilizing reaction of respiratory homeostasis*, and chronic allergic inflammation of the bronchi as **a part of the mechanism** of reversible bronchial obstruction known today.

CO_2-deficient theory of bronchial asthma by Dr K. Buteyko

A decrease in CO_2 in the lungs leads to an increase in uneven ventilation of the lungs and the appearance of symptoms of *bronchospasm*, which acts until the normalization of this *constant* and is able to be eliminated **by itself (automatically)** as *respiratory homeostasis* normalizes, which makes it possible to consider *bronchospasm* and reversible bronchial obstruction as a *homeostatic reaction of the functional respiratory system.*

Normalization of the CO_2 *constant* in the lungs leads to recovery or clinical remission of bronchial asthma, some cases of which have been observed for more than 50 years.

The theory was proposed by the Russian scientist Dr K. Buteyko (1923-2003) in the 1970s on the basis of his scientific discovery of *deep breathing disease.*

1. For the first time, the fundamental scientific research by Dr K. Buteyko established an inverse relationship between a decrease in CO_2 in the lungs and an increase in uneven ventilation of the lungs, which allows us today to consider reversible bronchial obstruction and *bronchospasm* as a *stabilizing reaction of respiratory homeostasis*, which occurs when the CO_2 *constant* in the lungs changes and is able to eliminate itself as it normalizes.

2. Scientific research by Dr K. Buteyko and long-term clinical practice have shown that clinical manifestations of bronchial asthma (cough, wheezing, whistling, suffocation) get stronger as *alveolar hypocapnia* increases, and also eliminate themselves as the CO_2 *constant* in the lungs is being normalized, which indicates an undoubted feedback between CO_2 in the lungs and chronic allergic inflammation of the bronchi.

3. Clinical manifestations of *bronchospasm* and *reversible bronchial obstruction* decrease and are eliminated by themselves as *alveolar hypocapnia* is eliminated and the CO_2 *constant* in the lungs is normalized, which makes it possible to consider allergic inflammation of the bronchi only as part of the mechanism of *reversible bronchial obstruction*, but **not as** its main cause.

4. Dr K. Buteyko pointed out that the cause of alveolar hypocapnia in asthma patients is chronic hyperventilation of the lungs (deep breathing), which increases as a result of forced inactivity and provokes bronchospasm, an attack of suffocation and all manifestations of reversible bronchial obstruction.

Dr K. Buteyko emphasized that forced *hypodynamia* (prolonged inactivity) in patients with asthma increases *hyperventilation of the lungs, alveolar hypocapnia* and manifestations of bronchial obstruction.

5. The drug-free method proposed by Dr K. Buteyko for the treatment of bronchial asthma, known as the Buteyko Method, uses three ways to normalize the CO_2 *constant* in the lungs and *respiratory homeostasis* in general:

- breathing techniques based on the principle of *gradually reducing the depth of breathing to normal*, which allows you to quickly eliminate the clinical manifestations of asthma;
- dosed physical (muscular) exercises under the control of breathing dynamics, which allows one to increase the activity of metabolism, normalize the CO_2 *constant* in the lungs and eliminate *metabolic hypoxia*;
- formation of a fine sensitivity to breathing, which allows a former asthma patient to monitor and understand changes in respiratory function in order to prevent *hyperventilation of the lungs* and changes in the CO_2 *constant* in the lungs.

Prevention of the recurrence of asthma or its exacerbations

Normalization of the CO_2 *constant* in the lungs using *the Buteyko Method* makes it possible to achieve recovery as *respiratory homeostasis* normalizes.

The maintaining of *respiratory homeostasis*, with the help of regular exercises with simple physical exercises or elementary sports, can effectively prevent the recurrence of bronchial asthma or its exacerbations during Buteyko treatment and recovery.

Why it is impossible to cure asthma completely with medication

Today, according to the generally accepted theory of bronchial asthma, the main clinical manifestation of this disease is *reversible bronchial obstruction*, which occurs as a result of *chronic allergic inflammation of the bronchi* and completely depends on its activity.

The cause and mechanism of *allergic inflammation of the bronchi* are not known, but it is believed that to eliminate asthma, it is necessary to eliminate this inflammation.

An effective treatment is corticosteroids, which reduce inflammation of the bronchi, which allows you to 'control asthma'.

Neither corticosteroids nor other known medications can eliminate *chronic allergic inflammation of the bronchi* **completely**, so it is impossible to cure asthma completely with medications.

Why the Buteyko Method completely cures bronchial asthma

It should be remembered that Dr K. Buteyko's scientific research has shown an undoubted relationship between the intensity of *allergic inflammation of the bronchi* and the pressure of CO_2 in the lungs *(pCO_2)*, which makes it possible to eliminate bronchial asthma **completely**, provided that the CO_2 *constant* in the lungs is normalized.

Deep breathing disease

The clinical manifestation of *homeostatic (stabilizing) reactions of the functional respiratory system* and other organism systems, from metabolic to behavioural, the normal operation of which is functionally related to the respiratory system.

Elements of the theory of deep breathing disease (according to Dr K. Buteyko)

1. The fundamental scientific research by Dr K. Buteyko was the development of the theory of the Russian physiologist, academician, Professor Peter K. Anokhin, according to which the human organism, as an *open*

system, is able to maintain the constancy of the internal environment - *homeostasis*, thanks to the work of a large complex of self-organizing and self-regulating physiological *functional systems of the organism*. Each of them maintains appropriate physiological *constants* (organism temperature, blood pressure, blood sugar, blood oxygen and many others), which ensures normal functioning and adaptation to changing environmental conditions.

A change in vital *constants* and a violation of *homeostasis* leads to the emergence of homeostatic (stabilizing) reactions of the corresponding physiological *functional systems of the organism*, which act before the normalization of *constants* and are able to eliminate themselves as *homeostasis* normalizes.

2. Dr K. Buteyko emphasized that homeostatic reactions form the clinical picture of diseases of organs and systems, often anatomically unrelated, but taking part in the construction of *the functional system of the organism*.

The physiology of *the functional systems of the organism* unites individual organs into systems not according to anatomical features and location, as is customary in classical physiology, but according to the tasks for which such an association of systems and organs is intended.

For example, *respiration* is a gas exchange between the cells of the organism and atmospheric air. To maintain *constant* values of respiratory gases in the cell (oxygen - O_2, carbon dioxide - CO_2), a *functional respiratory system* was formed, consisting of an external respiratory system (lung ventilation) and a transport system for respiratory gases (circulatory system).

A change in the *constants* of CO_2 or O_2 in cells, in the blood or in the lungs activates the corresponding *homeostatic (stabilizing) reactions of the functional respiratory system*.

For example, the inverse relationship discovered by Dr K. Buteyko between a decrease in CO_2 in the alveoli of the lungs and the appearance of symptoms of *bronchospasm*, as well as an increase in blood pressure during the development of *metabolic hypoxia*, make it possible to consider both *bronchospasm* and arterial hypertension as a stabilizing reaction of respiratory homeostasis. The proof is the ability of both *bronchospasm* and

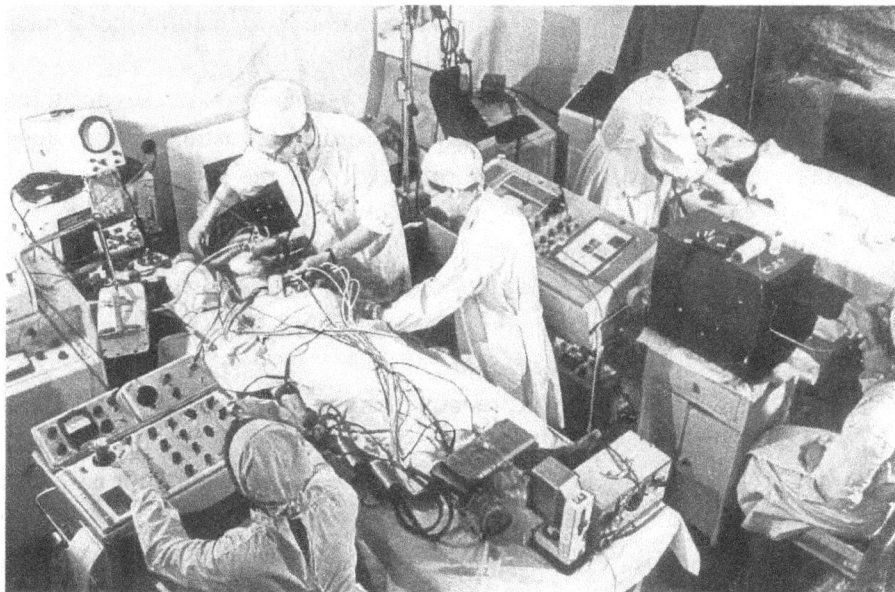

10. Dr K. Buteyko in the Laboratory of Functional Diagnostics, Institute of Experimental Biology and Medicine of the USSR Academy of Sciences, Novosibirsk, 1970s

arterial hypertension to be eliminated by themselves as *respiratory homeostasis* and the corresponding gas *constants* normalize.

3. Dr K. Buteyko pointed out that *hyperventilation of the lungs (deep breathing)* does not increase the supply of oxygen to arterial blood, which is always and under any conditions completely *saturated* with oxygen. But hyperventilation of the lungs is the cause of CO_2 deficiency in the lungs *(alveolar hypocapnia)*, the cause of CO_2 deficiency in arterial blood *(arterial hypocapnia)*, which, according to *the Verigo-Bohr effect*, hinders the transfer of oxygen from arterial blood to cells and creates *metabolic hypoxia. Hyperventilation of the lungs (deep breathing)* is ultimately the cause of oxygen deficiency in the cells.

4. Consistently occurring *alveolar hypocapnia, arterial hypocapnia* and *metabolic hypoxia* trigger *homeostatic (stabilizing) reactions of the functional respiratory system* with the development of reversible *bronchial*

obstruction, bronchospasm, arterial hypertension, which form the clinical picture of the corresponding diseases.

5. Dr K. Buteyko pointed out that the treatment of diseases resulting from the action of homeostatic reactions (bronchial asthma, high blood pressure) should be based on the normalization of the corresponding *constants*, which clinically always leads to recovery.

6. Drug treatment or low efficiency of homeostatic reactions is the cause of the transition of reversible functional disorders (*bronchospasm*) into organic damage (pneumofibrosis, atherosclerosis), which should also be considered as homeostatic reactions.

For example, regular use of bronchodilators to eliminate *bronchospasm* reduces its effectiveness as a homeostatic mechanism based on functional, reversible changes and leads to the emergence of pneumofibrosis as a homeostatic mechanism based on irreversible organic damage.

The causes of deep breathing disease

Dr K. Buteyko distinguished two causes of *deep breathing disease*:

- the main cause is the *hypodynamia (*prolonged inactivity) and decreased metabolic activity;
- *chronic hyperventilation of the lungs (deep breathing)* with the development of *alveolar hypocapnia, metabolic hypoxia* and violation of *respiratory homeostasis*.

Hypodynamia is indicated as the main cause of deep breathing disease, because a sufficient amount of muscle activity (sports or any physical activity) is a natural mechanism for the normalization of *gas constants* and *respiratory homeostasis*.

Hyperventilation of the lungs or 'deep breathing'

This means a pathological increase in general ventilation of the lungs under the condition of unchanged metabolic activity.

The chronic form of *hyperventilation of the lungs* is characterized by alveolar hyperventilation with the development of *alveolar hypocapnia, metabolic hypoxia,* violation of *respiratory homeostasis* and the occurrence of *homeostatic (stabilizing) reactions of the functional respiratory system,* the effect of which is aimed at normalizing gas *constants* and *respiratory homeostasis.*

The effect of *homeostatic reactions of the functional respiratory system* and other systems, the normal operation of which is functionally related to breathing, forms the clinical picture of *deep breathing disease.*

Graphic recording of breathing in patients with *chronic hyperventilation of the lungs* (bronchial asthma, allergies, high blood pressure, snoring, sleep apnea, chronic fatigue, and others) shows an increase in **the depth** of breathing with a slight change in other parameters, so Dr K. Buteyko suggested using the phrase *'deep breathing'* to denote *chronic hyperventilation of the lungs.* (Dr K. Buteyko, 'Regulation of bronchial tone in healthy and patients with bronchial asthma'. Institute of Physiology, Siberian Branch of the USSR Academy of Sciences, Novosibirsk, Akademgorodok, 1967, manuscript)

Hypodynamia (Physical inactivity)

The reduction of muscular (physical) activity to two or less hours a day as a result of a sedentary lifestyle.

It is characterized by a decrease in the activity of the general metabolism, a decrease in CO_2 production, as a result of which normal ventilation of the lungs, during which CO_2 is removed, becomes excessive due to CO_2 deficiency.

Dr K. Buteyko points to inactivity as the main cause of *deep breathing disease,* because muscle activity is a natural mechanism for normalization of gas *constants.*

Normalization of the CO_2 constant during elementary sports and other types of muscular activity normalizes oxygen supply to cells and eliminates *metabolic hypoxia.*

Dr K. Buteyko argued that the clinical manifestation of *deep breathing disease* depends on the type of homeostatic reactions of various levels seeking to normalize *respiratory homeostasis*, and the effectiveness of treatment depends on the ability to normalize the corresponding *constants*.

For example, normalization of the CO_2 *constant* in the lungs using *the Buteyko Method* makes it possible to eliminate *bronchospasm* without medication, while the use of bronchodilators reduces the effectiveness of *bronchospasm* as a functional, reversible homeostatic reaction, which will lead to the development of pneumofibrosis, which should also be considered as a homeostatic reaction, the effect of which is based on an irreversible reduction in the area of gas exchange as a result of organic damage to the lung tissue.

Treatment of *bronchospasm* and prevention of pneumofibrosis are possible only with normalization of the CO_2 *constant* in the lungs.

Hyperventilation syndrome

A set of symptoms resulting from *chronic hyperventilation of the lungs,* prolonged inactivity, changes in gas *constants* in the lungs, blood, cells and the action of homeostatic (stabilizing) reactions seeking to normalize *constants* and *respiratory homeostasis*.

For example, *bronchospasm* resulting from a change in the CO_2 *constant* in the lungs or an increase in blood pressure as a result of O_2 deficiency in cells are clinical manifestations of hyperventilation syndrome and *deep breathing disease*.

The therapeutic principle of the Buteyko Method

This is a gradual reducing of the depth of breathing to normal.

1. Graphic recording of breathing in patients with *chronic hyperventilation of the lungs* shows an increase in **the depth** of breathing with a slight change in other parameters, on the basis of which Dr K. Buteyko for the first time used the principle of gradually reducing the depth of breathing to normal and created a drug-free method of treatment known as *the Buteyko Method*.

Dr K. Buteyko repeatedly stressed that an arbitrary change in other parameters of the breathing pattern does not allow one to get a therapeutic result. Breathing techniques based on the principle of gradually reducing the depth of breathing to normal allow you to normalize the gas *constants* in the respiratory system and eliminate the vivid symptoms of the disease without the use of drugs.

2. To eliminate *hypodynamia* as the main cause of *deep breathing disease*. Dr K. Buteyko for the first time suggested using physical exercises with the control of breathing, which allows one to quickly normalize metabolic activity and normalize *respiratory homeostasis* no matter the disease.

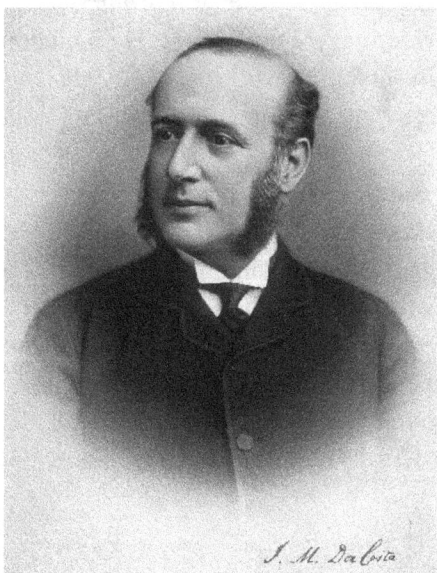

The history of the discovery of the 'deep breathing' disease

More than 100 years ago, during the American Civil War, an American doctor and surgeon, Professor Jacob Da Costa (Jacob Mendes Da Costa, 1833-1900), drew attention to visually noticeable and very deep breathing in veterans who complained of heart rhythm disorders, sleep disorders, persistent feeling of lack of air, panic attacks, nervous disorders and claimed the existence of hyperventilation syndrome.

11. Jacob Mendes Da Costa, 1833-1900

However, it was not possible to prove from a scientific point of view the connection of deep breathing of veterans with the development of these diseases at that time.

A hundred years later, in the 1970s, the Russian doctor and scientist Konstantin Pavlovich Buteyko (1923-2003) conducted fundamental scientific research on the physiology of respiration and proved the connection of *hyperventilation of the lungs* with the development of characteristic symptoms.

Dr K. Buteyko for **the first time** declared the existence of *deep breathing disease*, and also **explained the mechanism** of its development.

He **offered a scientifically based** method of treatment named *the Buteyko Method*. Dr K. Buteyko suggested using the term 'deep breathing' to refer to *chronic hyperventilation of the lungs*. He included *hyperventilation syndrome,* discovered by Professor Jacob Da Costa (Jacob Mendes Da Costa) in the composition of *deep breathing disease* and said, "I own the second part of a fundamental scientific discovery: I discovered and proved the existence of *deep breathing disease*, deciphered the mechanism of action of *deep breathing* on the human organism and invented a way to treat *deep breathing disease*." (Dr K. Buteyko, lecture at the city polyclinic No. 137, Moscow, 1979, transcript of the audio recording, manuscript)

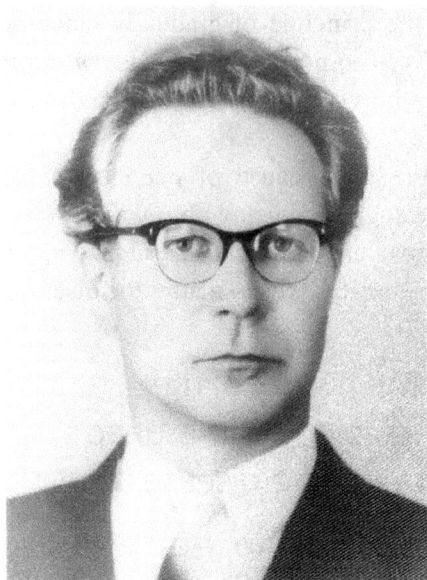

12. Dr K. Buteyko, 7 October 1952, on the date of his scientific discovery

Elements of the theory of degradation and death of modern civilization (according to Dr K. Buteyko)

1. Dr K. Buteyko argued that *deep breathing disease*, creating chronic hypoxia of the cerebral cortex responsible for intellectual (reasonable) activity, is the reason for the predominance of subcortical instincts characteristic of animal behaviour (sexual, food and others) in human behaviour.

2. The predominance of subcortical (animal) instincts turns reasonable human activity for learning and development of the surrounding world into aggressive and destructive behaviour, which will inevitably lead to the

death of civilization as a result of poisoning the habitat or its destruction (industrial chemistry, herbicides, antibiotics, wars, etc.).

3. *Deep breathing disease* is the cause of the mass spread of so-called diseases of civilization: allergies, bronchial asthma, high blood pressure, atherosclerosis and others.

4. Modern civilization has a planetary character; therefore, the death of civilization on the scale of all the planets threatens the existence of humanity as a biological species.

Functional system of the organism

The physiological functional system of the organism is a self-organizing and self-regulating complex of individual components, whose mutual activity is aimed at achieving an adaptive result, useful for the organism in order to adapt to the environment.

The Russian scientist, physiologist and academician, Professor Peter K. Anokhin, proposed a theory according to which the human organism is a complex of self-organizing and self-regulating functional systems, the normal operation of which ensures the maintenance of constant physiological values - *constants*, which allow the organism, as *an open system,* to maintain the constancy of the internal environment of the organism – *homeostasis*, and to adapt to changing environmental conditions.

The organism as an open system

The human organism is a so-called *open system,* which is affected by numerous external environmental factors, but which nevertheless maintains the constancy of its internal environment, or *homeostasis*, which is a condition for normal functioning and adaptation of the organism to its environment.

The normal operation of the entire complex of functional systems of the organism ensures *homeostasis* and *health*.

For example, the organism's temperature of 36.6 degrees is a constant value, a *constant*; blood pressure of 120/80 mm Hg is a *constant*; blood sugar of 5 mmol/liter is a *constant*; and many other *constants* that are supported by the work of numerous functional systems provide in total the constancy of the internal environment of the organism and our *health*.

Physiology of functional systems of the organism

The physiology of the functional systems of the organism unites individual organs into systems, not according to anatomical features and location, as is customary in classical physiology, but according to the tasks for which such an association of systems and organs is intended.

For example, the *functional respiratory system* provides gas exchange between the cells of the organism and the atmosphere (respiration).

To maintain the vital constants of oxygen (O_2) and carbon dioxide (CO_2) in the cells of the organism, a functional respiratory system has been formed, which consists of an *external respiration system* (lung ventilation) and transport for respiratory gases (circulatory system).

In this case, anatomically different formations - the respiratory organs and the circulatory system - are combined into a functional system to perform a common task - maintaining the *constants* of CO_2 and O_2 and *respiratory homeostasis* - the constancy of the gas composition of blood and cells.

Self-regulation of the physiological functional system

This is the mechanism for returning the deviated function to the initial level, to the level of normal vital activity and optimal cellular metabolism.

The mechanism of self-regulation forms *stabilizing (homeostatic) reactions of the functional systems of the organism*, which arise when *constants* change and are eliminated themselves as *homeostasis* normalizes.

For example, when gas *constants* change, *stabilizing (homeostatic) reactions of the functional respiratory system* are formed, which aim at normalizing *constants* and *respiratory homeostasis*.

Scientific research by Dr K. Buteyko has shown an undoubted inverse relationship between the decrease of CO_2 in the lungs and the appearance of symptoms of *bronchospasm*, which allows us to consider *bronchospasm* as a mechanism for normalization of the CO_2 *constant* in the lungs.

Health

This is a condition in which all vital *constants* are within the physiological norm as a result of the normal operation of the corresponding physiological functional systems of the organism.

Disease

This is a clinical manifestation of *homeostatic (stabilizing) reactions of functional systems of the organism* at various levels, from metabolic to behavioural, the action of which seeks to normalize physiological *constants* and *homeostasis*.

The further the *constants* have shifted from the normal level, the more *homeostatic (stabilizing) mechanisms* are involved and the disease is more severe.

For example, in patients with mild asthma, *hyperventilation of the lungs* and a change in the CO_2 *constant* are the cause of *bronchospasm*, which is able to eliminate itself as this *constant* gets normalized in the lungs.

The inverse relationship discovered by Dr K. Buteyko between CO_2 pressure in the lungs and bronchial tone in diseases occurring with increased bronchial tone allows us to consider *bronchospasm* as a mechanism for normalizing the CO_2 *constant* in the lungs, which has a functional, reversible character and is not accompanied by organic damage.

The use of bronchodilators reduces the effectiveness of *bronchospasm* as a functional (reversible) homeostatic reaction, which leads to severe asthma with pneumofibrosis, which should also be considered as a homeostatic reaction. Its effect is accompanied by irreversible damage to the lungs in order to reduce the gas exchange area to normalize the CO_2 *constant*.

Diagnostics

This means the search for *constants* that have gone beyond the norm and the physiological *functional system of the organism*, the work of which is disrupted.

Treatment

This is the process of normalization of the key parameters of homeostasis through exposure directly to a *constant* or to a *functional system of the organism* whose operation maintains this *constant* within the normal range.

Prevention

This means the prevention of displacement of *constants* beyond the limits of the norm.

Homeostasis

This is the constancy of the internal environment of the organism, from the ancient Greek meaning 'the same' or 'immobility'.

The dynamic balance between the disturbing effect and the response *stabilizing (homeostatic) reaction of the organism* allows to maintain *constants* (temperature, oxygen, CO_2, salts, and many others) within normal limits and within very strict limits.

Constant

This is a parameter whose value does not change.

Homeostatic constant

This is a constant parameter supported by the work of the corresponding *functional system of the organism* or homeostatic system. When the constant changes, stabilizing (homeostatic) reactions of the corresponding functional system are formed in order to normalize the constant.

Homeostatic (stabilizing) reaction of the functional system

This is the response of the *functional system of the organism* aiming at normalization of the changed key *constant* of *homeostasis*.

The Russian physiologist and academician, Professor Peter K. Anokhin, proposed a theory according to which the human organism is a so-called *open system* in which homeostasis maintains the constancy of the internal environment due to the work of a complex of self-organizing and self-regulating functional systems. This complex ensures the adaptation of the organism to changing environmental conditions.

Each physiological *functional system of the organism* maintains certain *constants* (organism temperature, blood pressure, blood sugar, electrolytes, oxygen and many others), the totality of which creates *homeostasis* and ensures *health*.

Changing the *constants* activates homeostatic (stabilizing) reactions of the corresponding *functional systems of the organism* in order to normalize them.

The physiology of *the functional systems of the organism* unites individual organs into systems, not according to anatomical features and location, as is customary in classical physiology, but according to the tasks for which such an association of systems and organs is intended.

For example, in order to maintain *constant* values of respiratory gases (O_2, CO_2) in the cells, the blood and the lungs, a *functional respiratory system* was formed, consisting of an external respiratory system (lung ventilation) and a transport system for respiratory gases (circulatory system).

A change in *constants* at any level causes a stabilizing reaction of the *functional respiratory system* with the development of corresponding diseases: a change in the CO_2 *constant* in the lungs causes *bronchospasm* with an outcome in bronchial asthma; a change in the O_2 *constant* in the cell causes an increase in blood pressure and hypertension.

The effective operation of the stabilizing reaction normalizes *constants* and limits the manifestations of the disease only to functional (reversible) disorders.

Low efficiency or drug elimination of homeostatic reactions leads to irreversible organic damage and a severe form of the disease.

For example, frequent use of bronchodilators reduces the effectiveness of *bronchospasm* as a reversible homeostatic reaction and leads to the rapid development of pneumofibrosis, which should also be considered as a homeostatic reaction, the effect of which is based on an irreversible reduction in the area of gas exchange. Therefore effective treatment of *bronchospasm* and prevention of pneumofibrosis are possible only as the CO_2 *constant* in the lungs normalizes.

Respiratory homeostasis

This is constancy of the gas composition of blood and tissues.

It is ensured by the normal operation of *the functional respiratory system*, which maintains gas *constants* (carbon dioxide - CO_2, oxygen - O_2) in the lungs, the blood and cells within the physiological norm.

The movement of respiratory gases (CO_2, O_2) is the main regulator of acid-base equilibrium (pH).

A change in gas *constants* at any level (in the lungs, the blood and cells) disrupts respiratory homeostasis and activates stabilizing (homeostatic) reactions, the clinical manifestations of which are *bronchial obstruction, bronchospasm* and pneumofibrosis, arterial hypertension, cholesterol and atherosclerosis, with the development of corresponding diseases.

Metabolic hypoxia

This is lack of oxygen (O_2) in cells, at the level of metabolism.

It occurs as a result of *chronic hyperventilation of the lungs (deep breathing)*, and largely forms the clinical picture of *deep breathing disease*.

It is a violation of *respiratory homeostasis*, which leads to a violation of metabolism, immunity and the formation of *homeostatic (compensatory) reactions of the functional systems of the organism*, with the development of corresponding diseases.

It is the cause of chronic fatigue, attention deficit, cognitive decline, poor exercise tolerance, severe pregnancy and childbirth, complications in the postpartum period, poor tissue regeneration and other manifestations of *deep breathing disease*.

Minute volume of breathing

The physiological parameter that allows us to evaluate lung ventilation is measured in litres per minute and shows the amount of air that passes through the lungs for one minute.

In the process of breathing and ventilation of the lungs, carbon dioxide is removed and oxygen enters the arterial blood.

Our organism is a so-called *open system* that communicates with the environment and is influenced by numerous environmental factors. Nevertheless, the organism maintains the constancy of its own internal environment - *homeostasis*.

Numerous *functional systems of the organism* maintain many constant values - *physiological constants*, which together provide *homeostasis* and are a condition for the normal functioning of the organism. For example, despite changing external conditions and environmental influences, our organism maintains a constant organism temperature, constant blood pressure, constant blood sugar, constant oxygen in the blood, and so on. All these numerous parameters are physiological *constants* that are maintained within a very narrow framework by various *functional systems of the organism*, which ensure our *health*.

Oxygen and carbon dioxide are physiological *constants*, the maintenance of which in the lungs, the blood and cells is provided by the *functional respiratory system*.

Respiration is the process of gas exchange between the cells of the organism and atmospheric air.

The cells of our organism receive oxygen from the atmospheric air, while CO_2 is formed in the cells as a result of metabolism, enters the blood and is removed from the organism during lung ventilation.

If the ventilation of the lungs exceeds the activity of metabolism, then a deficiency of CO_2 in the lungs and arterial blood develops (the initial stage of *deep breathing disease*), as well as a deficiency of oxygen at the metabolic level, at the cellular level, which leads to the formation of *homeostatic reactions of the functional respiratory system*, which normalize gas *constants* and form the clinical picture of *deep breathing disease*.

Dr K. Buteyko discovered the *deep breathing disease*, the theory of which goes back to the fundamental scientific research of the Russian physiologist I. M. Sechenov and the Russian academician of medicine, Professor P. K. Anokhin, who created the theory of *functional systems of the organism*.

Dr K. Buteyko published elements of the theory of *deep breathing disease* in the article 'Ventilation test in patients with bronchial asthma' (*Medical Work*, 1968, No. 4, Institute of Physiology of the Academy of Medical Sciences of the USSR):

- under normal conditions, arterial blood is always completely saturated with oxygen;
- an arbitrary increase in lung ventilation does not increase oxygen in arterial blood;
- an arbitrary change in the minute volume of respiration or general ventilation of the lungs using various breathing techniques does not increase or decrease oxygen in arterial blood;
- under normal conditions, an arbitrary increase in lung ventilation with unchanged metabolic activity is the cause of CO_2 deficiency in the lungs (*alveolar hypocapnia*) and arterial blood (*arterial hypocapnia*), as well as subsequent oxygen deficiency in cells - *metabolic hypoxia (Verigo-Bohr effect)*;
- the functional respiratory system reacts to changes in the CO2 constant and normalizes it much faster than the O2 constant, which indicates the

priority of the CO2 constant for the normal functioning of the organism;
- excessive respiration *(hyperventilation of the lungs)* and subsequent oxygen deficiency in cells *(metabolic hypoxia)* are the cause of the formation of *homeostatic reactions of the functional respiratory system*, the action of which is aimed at normalizing the constants of CO2 and O2. *Homeostatic reactions* form the clinical picture of the corresponding diseases: for example, chronic rhinitis or *reversible bronchial obstruction* occur when the *constant* of CO2 in the lungs changes, act until its partial or complete normalization and are able to be eliminated automatically as *respiratory homeostasis* normalizes.

Peripheral vasodilation

This is an increase in the diameter of peripheral blood vessels as a result of a decrease in the tone of the vascular wall.

It occurs as a result of normalization of oxygen *constants* (O_2) in cells and CO_2 in arterial blood using *the Buteyko Method*, which makes it possible to effectively treat hypertension, vegetative-vascular dystonia and a number of diseases occurring with peripheral angiospasm.

Peripheral angiospasm

A spasm (compression) of peripheral blood vessels, resulting in an increase in blood pressure *(arterial hypertension)*.

According to the theory of *deep breathing disease* proposed by the Russian physiologist and physician Dr K. Buteyko, peripheral angiospasm is a *homeostatic reaction of the functional respiratory system*, which is formed as a result of *metabolic hypoxia* (oxygen deficiency in cells, in metabolism) and is confirmed by its ability to eliminate itself as the normalization of the O_2 *constant* in cells, the CO_2 *constant* in arterial blood and *respiratory homeostasis* occurs.

Deep breathing, creating a deficiency of CO_2 in arterial blood, prevents the transfer of oxygen from the blood to the cells *(the Verigo-Bohr effect)* and is the cause of *metabolic hypoxia* and *respiratory homeostasis* disorders.

Peripheral angiospasm and arterial hypertension, which have arisen in order to eliminate *metabolic hypoxia*, are functional (reversible) homeostatic reactions, the low efficiency of which may cause an increase in cholesterol and the development of atherosclerosis of blood vessels, which should be considered as organic (irreversible) homeostatic reactions of the physiological *functional respiratory system*.

The medical technology created by Dr K. Buteyko, known as *the Buteyko Method,* makes it possible to cure diseases without drugs that occur with an increase in blood pressure, an increase in cholesterol and the development of atherosclerosis of blood vessels.

Saturation

This is about saturation of arterial blood with oxygen during respiration, during lung ventilation.

Normally, under any conditions, saturation is 93-98%, except for diseases with a decrease in the area of gas exchange (prolonged bronchial spasm, pneumofibrosis).

It is important to remember that ventilation of the lungs is always carried out evenly over the entire surface of the lungs. Slightly less according to anatomical features are ventilated the tops of the lungs in a horizontal position.

No breathing techniques, no breathing exercises or simulators are capable of improving or increasing the uniformity of lung ventilation or lung volume, except for *chronic hyperventilation of the lungs*.

Hyperventilation of the lungs, creating a shortage of CO_2, leads to a violation of the uniformity of lung ventilation and the appearance of clinical signs of *bronchial obstruction and bronchospasm* in 30% of the population. They disrupt air access to the gas exchange zone in the lungs and it leads to the diminishing of gas exchange surface, which in turn can affect arterial blood saturation according to the indication of a simple pulse oximeter.

Ignoring the fact that lung ventilation is always carried out evenly over the entire pulmonary surface, as well as the fact that arterial blood is always 93-98% saturated with oxygen under any conditions, generates a lot of ridiculous, monstrous breathing exercises and breathing simulators in order to 'make work lungs after illness' or 'increase oxygen entry'.

20% of the remaining lungs after pneumonia are able to provide 95% saturation in the absence of hyperventilation of the lungs or mechanical ventilation

The Covid-19 pandemic has shown that an 80% reduction in the area of gas exchange in the lungs after pneumonia does not significantly affect arterial blood saturation.

To maintain normal saturation (95%), 20% of the normal lung volume is sufficient with normal air access to the gas exchange zone in the lungs (absence of *bronchial obstruction*).

The use of mechanical lung ventilation (ventilator) in the mode of *hyperventilation of the lungs* (excessive ventilation and positive pressure at the end of exhalation) in order to increase arterial blood saturation gives the opposite result and is often the main cause of death of the patient:

1. *Hyperventilation of the lungs* on a ventilator leads to a deficiency of CO_2 in the lungs *(alveolar hypocapnia)*, in the blood *(arterial hypocapnia)* and, according to *the Verigo-Bohr effect*, a deficiency of oxygen in metabolism *(metabolic hypoxia)*;

2. In diseases with a large area of lung destruction (for example, pneumonia with Covid-19), an increase in CO_2 deficiency in the lungs in 30% of cases is the cause of bronchial obstruction (bronchial edema, sputum hypersecretion, bronchospasm), which makes it difficult for air to reach intact areas of the lungs;

3. A decrease in the area of gas exchange in the lungs does not allow the effective removal of excess CO_2 from the venous blood, which leads to blood shunting and *arterial hypercapnia*, which may cause the death of the patient.

Metabolic hypoxia may occur with normal saturation

Normal saturation is not an indicator of normal gas exchange in tissues and cells, at the level of metabolism.

The supply of oxygen from arterial blood to cells does not depend on the saturation of arterial blood, but on the pressure of CO_2 (pCO_2).

With the development of CO_2 deficiency, it is difficult to transfer oxygen from the blood to the cells *(the Verigo-Bohr effect)*, which leads to *metabolic hypoxia* and the occurrence of corresponding diseases (post-Covid syndrome and post-Covid tachycardia, chronic fatigue, visual impairment, metabolic and immune disorders, etc.).

Treatment of post-Covid syndrome by the Buteyko Method

For the treatment of post-Covid syndrome, it is necessary to normalize *gas constants*: first of all the CO_2 *constant* in the lungs and arterial blood, on which the oxygen supply to the metabolism and the successful treatment of post-Covid syndrome depend.

Post-Covid tachycardia, chronic fatigue, visual impairment and all other manifestations of the so-called post-Covid syndrome are just vivid manifestations of *metabolic hypoxia*, oxygen deficiency in metabolism.

To eliminate *metabolic hypoxia*, it is necessary to normalize the CO_2 *constant* in the lungs and arterial blood using *the Buteyko Method*.

Influence of breathing techniques of the Buteyko Method on saturation

1. In the absence of bronchopulmonary diseases and normal lung function, the pulse oximeter shows a slight fluctuation in saturation from 95% to 100% with an arbitrary change in lung ventilation using various breathing techniques of *the Buteyko Method*.

2. In diseases occurring with increased bronchial tone and reversible decrease in the gas exchange area in the lungs (all diseases with *reversible*

bronchial obstruction and *bronchospasm*), always and regardless of the type of respiratory techniques of *the Buteyko Method,* the pulse oximeter shows an increase in saturation to normal values as a result of improved airway patency and air access to the gas exchange zone.

3. In diseases that occur with an irreversible decrease in the area of gas exchange (pneumofibrosis, lung destruction in Covid-19), the pulse oximeter in all cases demonstrates normalization of saturation, but in some cases with a significant fluctuation of the indicator (reduction to 80% or lower during the performance of certain types of Buteyko breathing techniques) with its rapid normalization (instantaneous increase to 100% after the first normal inhalation).

Verigo–Bohr effect

This is the dependence of oxyhemoglobin dissociation on the partial pressure of carbon dioxide *(pCO₂)* in the lungs and arterial blood.

A decrease in carbon dioxide due to *hyperventilation of the lungs* or *hypodynamia* hinders the transfer of oxygen from the blood to the cells, which causes *metabolic hypoxia.*

The effect was discovered by the Russian physiologist Professor Bronislav F. Verigo in 1898 and rediscovered by the Danish physiologist Christian Bohr in 1904.

Dr K. Buteyko pointed out that, according to the Verigo-Bohr effect, *deep breathing* and prolonged inactivity (*hypodynamia)* are the cause of oxygen deficiency in metabolism *(metabolic hypoxia).*

Because of *deep breathing*, the occurred oxygen deficiency and violation of *respiratory homeostasis* are the cause of the formation of *homeostatic reactions of the functional respiratory system* (reversible reduction of the diameter of the respiratory tract and vascular spasm) with the development of corresponding diseases (bronchial obstruction and asthma, hypertension, high cholesterol, atherosclerosis).

pO$_2$, pCO$_2$

The partial pressure of oxygen and carbon dioxide. It is measured in the lungs and blood in millimeters of mercury (mm Hg) or volume percentages.

Maintenance of pCO$_2$, pO$_2$ and acid-base equilibrium (pH) is the main task of the physiological *functional system of respiration*. The movement of respiratory gases (O$_2$, CO$_2$) is the main regulator of pH.

The partial pressure of carbon dioxide (pCO$_2$), partial pressure of oxygen (pO$_2$) and acid-base equilibrium (pH) are vital constants whose normal values ensure health.

Dr K. Buteyko emphasized that the sensitivity of the *functional respiratory system* to the change in pCO$_2$ is ten times higher than the sensitivity to a change in pO$_2$.

A change in the CO$_2$ *constant* is the cause of the formation of *stabilizing reactions of the functional respiratory system*, the action of which normalize *constants* and *respiratory homeostasis*.

The clinical manifestation of stabilizing reactions of *respiratory homeostasis* are diseases with *bronchospasm* and *reversible bronchial obstruction*, pneumofibrosis, arterial hypertension, atherosclerosis.

Sapienti sat

Translating from the Latin: it is enough for the wise; the wise will understand; it is enough for understanding,

Titus Maccius Plautus, 3rd century BC